I0126402

Mental Health Nursing Essentials

A Simplified Guide for Students and New Nurses

Theo Seki

ISBN: 978-1-923370-58-6

Isohan Publishing

Table of Contents

Preface

Welcome. Stepping into the field of mental health nursing is unlike any other path in healthcare. It asks not only for your clinical skills—your assessment, your knowledge of medications, your ability to respond in a crisis—but also for your humanity. It requires you to connect with people experiencing profound distress, confusion, or despair, often related to experiences that challenge our very understanding of reality or endurance. It's demanding work, no question about it. It can push you, challenge your assumptions, and ask you to grow in ways you might not expect.

Yet, the rewards are equally profound. To witness someone, reclaim hope, to see understanding dawn in a family's eyes, to be a steady presence offering safety and respect when someone feels most lost—these are the moments that sustain us.

As a Registered Mental Nurse, I have seen firsthand the need for clear, practical guidance, especially for those just starting their journey—nursing students feeling overwhelmed by dense textbooks, or new graduates navigating the intense realities of clinical practice. Too often, essential knowledge feels buried in academic language or spread across too many sources.

This book, *Mental Health Nursing Essentials*, was born from that need. Its purpose is simple: to offer a **simplified, reader-friendly introduction** to the core concepts and skills required in psychiatric and mental health nursing. It's designed to be a **high-yield guide**, focusing on the essentials you truly need for exams and, more importantly, for providing safe, compassionate, and effective care.

We'll move through the foundations—understanding mental health and illness, the crucial therapeutic relationship, communication skills—and then explore common conditions like anxiety, depression, bipolar disorder, psychosis, personality disorders, substance use challenges, and the impact of trauma. We'll look at interventions, from pharmacology basics (demystified, I hope!) to other therapeutic approaches, always framing them within the structure of the nursing process. We will also touch upon the vital legal and ethical considerations that guide our practice, the importance of adapting care across the lifespan and diverse populations, and the non-negotiable necessity of caring for ourselves in this demanding field.

Throughout, you'll find case studies drawn from clinical reality (though altered to protect privacy), practical tips, memory aids, and key points highlighted. The aim is not to replace your comprehensive textbooks or experienced mentors, but to supplement them—to be a clear, accessible companion you can turn to for understanding and review.

Mental health nursing requires knowledge, skill, empathy, resilience, and perhaps above all, a genuine respect for the individuals we serve. It's my hope that this guide will provide you with a solid foundation and build your confidence as you embark on or continue this significant work. The journey requires dedication, but the difference you can make is immeasurable. Let's begin.

Theo Seki, RMN

Introduction

Why Mental Health Nursing Matters

Stepping into the world of mental health care is unlike entering any other area of nursing. It requires not just clinical skill but also a deep well of self-awareness, empathy, and a genuine desire to understand the human experience in all its variations. This isn't about fixing broken machines; it's about connecting with people during their most vulnerable times, helping them find strength, navigate challenges, and move toward recovery. You are entering a field where your presence, your words, and your understanding can be powerful agents of healing. It's demanding, yes, but the opportunity to witness resilience and facilitate meaningful change in people's lives is profoundly rewarding. Let's begin exploring what this unique specialty entails.

Welcome to the Field Its Importance and Scope

Mental health nursing—or psychiatric nursing, as it's often called—is a specialized field focused on the care of individuals, families, and communities experiencing mental health challenges or psychiatric disorders. But really, it's about promoting mental well-being for *everyone*. Think about it: there is no true health without mental health. Our minds and bodies are linked. Someone struggling with severe depression might neglect their physical health, just as someone managing chronic pain might develop anxiety. Mental health care isn't isolated; it's a fundamental part of holistic nursing practice.

The **importance** of this field cannot be overstated. Mental health conditions are common worldwide, affecting people of all ages, backgrounds, and walks of life. These conditions can impact thoughts, feelings, behaviors, and relationships, sometimes significantly disrupting daily life. Skilled, compassionate mental health nurses are essential for:

- Providing direct care and support.

- Helping individuals understand their conditions and treatment options.

- Administering medications safely and monitoring effects.

- Teaching coping skills and promoting resilience.

- Connecting people with resources.

- Advocating for patient rights and fighting stigma.

- Supporting families and caregivers.

The **scope** of mental health nursing is incredibly broad. You might picture nurses working solely in psychiatric hospitals, but that's just one piece of the picture. Mental health nurses practice in a wide array of settings:

- **Inpatient Psychiatric Units:** Providing acute care for individuals in crisis.

- **Community Mental Health Centers:** Offering ongoing support, therapy, and case management.

- **General Hospitals:** Working as consultation-liaison nurses, assisting medical teams with patients who have co-occurring mental health needs.

- **Substance Use Treatment Centers:** Helping individuals struggling with addiction and related mental health issues.

- **Forensic Settings:** Caring for individuals within the criminal justice system who have mental health conditions.

- **Schools and Universities:** Supporting students' mental well-being.

- **Private Practices:** Offering therapy and counseling.

- **Home Health Care:** Providing mental health support in patients' homes.

- **Telehealth:** Delivering care remotely via phone or video.

- **Military and Veterans Affairs:** Addressing the unique mental health needs of service members and veterans.

Case Study: The Unexpected Connection

- *Scenario:* Maria, a new RN on a busy medical-surgical floor, is caring for Mr. Henderson, a 68-year-old man recovering from pneumonia. His physical recovery is progressing, but Maria notices he's withdrawn, barely eats, often tearful, and makes comments like, "There's just no point anymore." His wife passed away six months ago. Other staff attribute his mood to being sick and hospitalized.*

- *Nurse's Action:* Maria recognizes these signs might indicate more than just situational sadness. During a quiet moment, she sits with Mr. Henderson, uses open-ended questions ("I've noticed you seem quite down lately, Mr. Henderson. Can you tell me more about what's been on your mind?"), and actively listens. He shares his profound grief, feelings of hopelessness, and lack of social support since his wife died. He admits he hasn't felt this way before his pneumonia. Maria validates his feelings ("It sounds incredibly difficult, losing your wife and now being unwell on top of that") and performs a basic depression screening, which indicates moderate to severe symptoms. She documents her findings and communicates her concerns to the medical team, specifically suggesting a consult with the psychiatric liaison nurse or mental health team.

- *Outcome:* The medical team, prompted by Maria's assessment, requests a psychiatric consultation. Mr. Henderson is diagnosed with Major Depressive Disorder, likely exacerbated by his grief and illness. He begins antidepressant medication and receives counseling from the liaison nurse. Maria continues to provide supportive care, encouraging him to eat, engage in small activities, and reinforcing the treatment plan. Upon discharge, he's connected with outpatient grief counseling and mental health services. Maria's attention to his *mental* health significantly impacted his overall recovery and well-being, demonstrating that mental health nursing principles are relevant everywhere.

This case shows how recognizing and addressing mental health needs is part of **all** nursing. Your skills in observation, communication, and assessment are applicable far beyond dedicated psychiatric settings.

Dispelling Myths and Reducing Stigma

One of the biggest hurdles in mental health care isn't a lack of treatments—it's **stigma**. Stigma refers to negative attitudes, beliefs, and discrimination directed towards people with mental health conditions. It creates an environment of shame, fear, and silence, preventing many from seeking the help they need. As nurses, we have a crucial role—an obligation, really—to challenge these harmful ideas.

Let's tackle some common **myths**:

- **Myth:** Mental illness is a sign of weakness or a character flaw.

- **Fact:** Mental illnesses are legitimate medical conditions, often involving biological, psychological, and social factors. They are illnesses, not choices or signs of poor character. Think of depression like diabetes or heart disease—it requires treatment and management.

- **Myth:** People with mental illness are violent and dangerous.

  - **Fact:** This is largely fueled by media sensationalism. The vast majority of people with mental illness are no more violent than the general population. In fact, they are more likely to be *victims* of violence than perpetrators. When violence does occur, it's often linked to other factors like substance use or lack of access to treatment, not solely the mental illness itself.

- **Myth:** People with mental illness can't recover or lead productive lives.

  - **Fact:** Recovery is possible and common! With appropriate treatment, support, and self-management strategies, many individuals with mental illness live full, meaningful, and productive lives. Recovery doesn't always mean the absence of symptoms, but rather living well *despite* them.

- **Myth:** You can just "snap out of" depression or anxiety.

  - **Fact:** Telling someone to "snap out of it" is like telling someone with a broken leg to just walk it off. Mental illnesses involve complex changes in brain chemistry, thought patterns, and emotional regulation that require professional help and support, not just willpower.

7

- **Myth:** Children don't experience mental health problems.
  - ○ **Fact:** Mental health conditions can begin in childhood or adolescence. Early identification and intervention are key to improving long-term outcomes. Conditions like anxiety, depression, ADHD, and behavioral disorders are diagnosed in young people.

Understanding Stigma:

Stigma operates on different levels:

1. **Public Stigma:** Negative attitudes held by the general public (e.g., believing people with schizophrenia are dangerous). This leads to discrimination in housing, employment, and social relationships.

2. **Self-Stigma:** When individuals internalize these negative public attitudes, leading to shame, low self-esteem, and reluctance to seek help ("Maybe they're right, maybe I *am* weak").

3. **Institutional Stigma:** Policies or practices within organizations (governments, healthcare systems, workplaces) that systematically disadvantage people with mental illness (e.g., inadequate insurance coverage for mental health care compared to physical health care).

The Nurse's Role in Reducing Stigma:

- **Educate:** Share accurate information about mental health with patients, families, colleagues, and the community. Correct misconceptions when you hear them.

- **Use Person-First Language:** Say "a person *with* schizophrenia" rather than "a schizophrenic." Focus on the person, not the diagnosis. Language shapes attitudes.

- **Be Mindful of Your Own Attitudes:** Examine your own beliefs and potential biases. Treat every individual with dignity and respect, regardless of their diagnosis.

- **Advocate:** Speak up for policies and practices that promote mental health equity and challenge discrimination. Support patient rights.

- **Promote Recovery:** Share stories of hope and recovery (while maintaining confidentiality). Emphasize strengths and resilience.

- **Provide Compassionate Care:** Your non-judgmental, empathetic approach can directly counteract the negative experiences many individuals have faced due to stigma.

Case Study: Overcoming Fear

- *Scenario:* David, a 24-year-old college student, experiences his first episode of psychosis, involving auditory hallucinations and paranoid thoughts. He is brought to the emergency department by his concerned roommate. David is terrified, not only by his symptoms but also by what this means. He grew up hearing relatives whisper about an uncle who was "crazy" and "locked away." He fears being judged, losing his friends, and being unable to finish his degree.*

- *Nurse's Action:* Sarah, the psychiatric nurse assessing David, approaches him calmly and introduces herself clearly. She avoids jargon. Instead of focusing immediately on the "psychosis," she asks about his *experience* — "It sounds like some really frightening things have been happening. Can you tell me what it's been like for you?" She listens without judgment as he haltingly describes the voices and his fears about people watching him. She normalizes seeking help: "Lots of people experience things like this, especially under stress. The important thing is that you're here now, and we can help figure out what's going on and how to make things better." She explains the assessment process simply and reassures him about confidentiality (within legal limits). She uses person-first language when documenting and speaking with the team. When David expresses fear about being "labeled crazy," Sarah responds, "We don't use labels like that here. We focus on understanding your symptoms and finding ways to help you feel safe and get back to your life. This is a health issue, like any other."

- *Outcome:* Sarah's approach helps reduce David's immediate fear and shame. He feels heard and respected, making him more willing to engage in further assessment and treatment planning. By directly addressing his fears related to stigma and modeling non-judgmental language and behavior, Sarah creates a therapeutic space that counteracts the negative messages David internalized. This interaction sets a positive tone for his subsequent care and his journey toward understanding and managing his condition.

Challenging stigma isn't just a nice thing to do; it's fundamental to effective mental health nursing. It opens doors for people to seek and accept help.

The Role of the Nurse in Mental Health Care

So, what does a mental health nurse actually *do*? The role is multifaceted, blending the art of human connection with the science of nursing. At its heart, it involves establishing **therapeutic relationships** built on trust, empathy, and respect. This relationship is the foundation upon which all other interventions are built.

Key responsibilities include:

1. **Assessment:** This is ongoing. It involves gathering information about the patient's mental and physical health, social situation, strengths, and challenges. This includes conducting the Mental Status Examination (MSE), risk assessments (suicide, self-harm, violence), understanding substance use patterns, and identifying coping mechanisms.

2. **Diagnosis:** While physicians or psychiatric nurse practitioners make medical diagnoses (like Schizophrenia or Bipolar Disorder), nurses formulate **nursing diagnoses**. These focus on the human *response* to health problems (e.g., *Ineffective Coping, Risk for Self-Directed Violence, Social Isolation, Disturbed Thought Processes*). Nursing diagnoses guide our care planning.

3. **Planning Care:** Working *collaboratively* with the patient (whenever possible), their family, and the interprofessional team (doctors, social workers, therapists, pharmacists, etc.), the nurse develops an individualized plan of care. This plan outlines specific goals and the nursing interventions needed to achieve them.

4. **Implementing Interventions:** This is where the nurse puts the plan into action. Interventions are diverse and require a broad skill set:

    o **Therapeutic Communication:** Using specific techniques to build rapport, encourage expression of feelings, challenge maladaptive thoughts, and provide support.

- o **Medication Administration and Management:** Safely giving medications, monitoring for effectiveness and side effects, and educating patients about their medications—this is a huge part of the role.

- o **Psychoeducation:** Teaching patients and families about mental health conditions, treatments, coping skills, relapse prevention, and available resources.

- o **Milieu Management:** Creating and maintaining a safe, therapeutic environment (the "milieu") on inpatient units or in group settings. This involves setting boundaries, managing group dynamics, and ensuring safety.

- o **Counseling and Support:** Providing supportive counseling, crisis intervention, and helping patients develop problem-solving skills.

- o **Promoting Self-Care Activities:** Assisting patients with activities of daily living (ADLs), hygiene, nutrition, sleep, and encouraging healthy habits.

- o **Behavioral Interventions:** Implementing strategies like behavior modification plans or token economies, often in collaboration with therapists.

5. **Evaluation:** Continuously evaluating the effectiveness of the care plan. Are the interventions working? Are the goals being met? Does the plan need to be adjusted? This involves ongoing assessment and critical thinking.

6. **Advocacy:** Being the voice for patients, ensuring their rights are protected, and helping them navigate the healthcare system. This might involve speaking up in team meetings, connecting patients with legal aid, or ensuring they understand their treatment options.

7. **Interprofessional Collaboration:** Mental health care is a team sport. Nurses work closely with psychiatrists, psychologists, social workers, occupational therapists, pharmacists, peer support specialists, and others to provide coordinated care.

8. **Therapeutic Use of Self:** This is perhaps the most unique aspect. It means consciously using your personality, insights, and judgments as part of the therapeutic process. It requires self-awareness—understanding your own feelings, biases, and how your presence affects others—and using that awareness to interact therapeutically.

Case Study: A Nurse's Day on the Unit

- *Scenario:* James is an RN working day shift on an acute inpatient psychiatric unit. His assignment includes four patients:

  - *Ms. A:* Admitted yesterday for severe depression and suicidal ideation. Requires close observation (15-minute checks).

  - *Mr. B:* Diagnosed with schizophrenia, experiencing auditory hallucinations and agitation. Needs PRN medication assessment.

  - *Ms. C:* Diagnosed with Bipolar I Disorder, currently manic, exhibiting pressured speech, poor boundaries, and intrusiveness with peers.

- Mr. D: Admitted for alcohol withdrawal, requiring vital sign monitoring and CIWA (Clinical Institute Withdrawal Assessment for Alcohol) scores.*

- *James's Actions & Thinking:*

  - *(Start of Shift):* Gets report, reviews orders and care plans. Prioritizes: Safety checks for Ms. A, vital signs/CIWA for Mr. D, assessing Mr. B's agitation.

  - *(7:30 AM):* Checks on Ms. A. Engages her briefly ("How was your night?"), observes her affect (flat), ensures she's safe. Documents check.

  - *(8:00 AM):* Assesses Mr. D – checks vital signs, performs CIWA. Notes mild tremors. Administers scheduled Librium per protocol. Provides reassurance.

  - *(8:30 AM):* Medication pass. Engages Ms. A again, encourages her to take her antidepressant. Assesses Mr. B – he reports "the voices are loud" and paces agitatedly. James uses calm communication, offers PRN antipsychotic, which Mr. B accepts. James monitors for effects. Engages Ms. C – redirects her gently but firmly when she interrupts another patient's conversation ("Ms. C, let's give Mr. X some space right now. Why don't we walk over here?"). Offers her scheduled mood stabilizer.

  - *(10:00 AM):* Attends interdisciplinary team meeting. Reports on his patients' progress, safety concerns (Ms. A), response to meds (Mr. B, Mr. D), and behavioral issues (Ms. C). Collaborates on adjustments to Ms. C's plan (suggesting structured activities to channel her energy).

Advocates for Ms. A to see the psychologist today.

- ○ *(Throughout Shift):* Conducts regular safety checks on Ms. A. Monitors Mr. B for medication effects and hallucination intensity. Redirects Ms. C multiple times, maintaining clear boundaries. Monitors Mr. D's withdrawal symptoms. Documents all assessments, interventions, and patient responses meticulously. Spends 1:1 time with Ms. A, using active listening while she talks about hopelessness. Teaches Mr. B a simple grounding technique for when voices are distressing. Encourages Ms. C to attend a group activity. Provides education to Mr. D about the withdrawal process.

- ○ *(End of Shift):* Completes final checks and documentation. Gives detailed report to the oncoming nurse.

- *Outcome:* James skillfully juggles multiple complex patients, constantly assessing, intervening, evaluating, and prioritizing safety. He uses therapeutic communication, medication management, milieu skills, and collaboration. His role isn't just task-based; it's about continuous therapeutic engagement and clinical judgment.

This example highlights the dynamic and demanding nature of the mental health nurse's role, requiring a blend of assessment skills, communication finesse, pharmacological knowledge, and strong interpersonal abilities.

How to Use This Guide Maximizing Your Learning

This guide is designed differently from your large, exhaustive textbooks. Think of it as a focused, practical companion for your mental health nursing journey. Our goal isn't to cover every single detail but to give you a solid grasp of the **essentials**—the core concepts, common conditions, key skills, and critical nursing considerations you *need* to know for exams and safe practice. It's deliberately simplified and high-yield.

To get the most out of this book:

1. **Focus on Understanding, Not Just Memorizing:** Don't just try to cram facts. Strive to understand the *why* behind concepts. Why is therapeutic communication important? Why do certain medications cause specific side effects? How does stigma impact care? Understanding leads to better retention and application.

2. **Engage with the Material Actively:**

    o Read the **case studies** carefully. Think about what *you* would do in that situation before reading the nurse's actions and outcomes. How does the case illustrate the chapter's concepts?

    o Pay attention to **bolded terms** and key concepts. Make sure you can define them in your own words.

    o Utilize the **tips, mnemonics, and quick reference** elements. These are designed as shortcuts to help you remember essential information.

    o Answer the **Practice Questions** at the end of each chapter. Don't just look up the answers—try to reason through them first. Read the **rationales** carefully, even for questions you got right. Understanding why an answer is correct (and why others are wrong) reinforces learning.

3. **Connect Theory to Practice:** As you read, think about patients you've encountered (or might encounter) in

clinical settings. How do these concepts apply to real people? If you're currently in a clinical rotation, try to link what you're learning here to your daily experiences.

4. **Use It as a Supplement:** This guide works well alongside your lectures and primary textbook. Use it to clarify confusing topics, review before exams, or quickly refresh your knowledge before a clinical shift. It provides a different, more streamlined perspective.

5. **Don't Skip the Foundational Chapters:** Understanding core concepts like the therapeutic relationship, communication, assessment, and stigma (like we covered here) is essential before moving on to specific disorders and interventions. These principles apply across the board.

6. **Reflect on Your Own Responses:** Mental health nursing often brings up personal feelings or biases. Pay attention to your reactions as you read. Self-awareness is a key nursing tool in this field.

This guide aims to be clear, practical, and supportive. It acknowledges that learning mental health nursing can feel overwhelming at first. By focusing on the essentials and presenting them in an accessible way, we hope to build your confidence and competence as you develop into a thoughtful and effective nurse, capable of making a real difference in the lives of those facing mental health challenges.

A Closing Reflection on Beginnings

We've laid some groundwork here, looking at the 'why' and 'what' of mental health nursing. It's a field brimming with challenges, yes, but also immense opportunities for connection and impact. Stepping into this requires shedding preconceived notions – both society's and sometimes our own – and embracing a perspective centered on the whole person and their unique journey toward well-being. The path ahead involves continuous learning, not just about disorders and treatments, but about ourselves and the profound therapeutic power of human presence.

Key Learnings from This Section

- **Mental Health is Foundational:** It's integral to overall health; mental health nursing addresses well-being and illness across diverse settings.

- **Stigma is a Major Barrier:** Negative myths and attitudes prevent help-seeking; nurses must actively combat stigma through education, language, and advocacy.

- **The Nurse's Role is Multifaceted:** Key functions include assessment (especially MSE), therapeutic communication, medication management, psychoeducation, milieu management, advocacy, and using the **therapeutic relationship** as the core tool.

- **Holistic Care is Essential:** Address the interconnected mental, physical, social, and spiritual needs of individuals.

- **Recovery is Possible:** Focus on hope, empowerment, and supporting individuals in living meaningful lives, even with ongoing symptoms.

- **Self-Awareness is Crucial:** Understanding your own responses and using your presence therapeutically is key (Therapeutic Use of Self).

- **This Guide is Focused:** Use it to grasp essential concepts, supplement learning, and prepare for practice with a high-yield approach.

Part 1: Foundations of Mental Health Nursing Practice

Chapter 1: Core Concepts and Frameworks Simplified

Before we can effectively nurse individuals experiencing mental health challenges, we need a shared understanding of some basic ideas. What exactly *is* mental health? How does it differ from mental illness? And how have our ways of thinking about these conditions developed? Understanding these core concepts isn't just academic—it directly shapes how you perceive your patients, how you interact with them, and the kind of care you provide. It's about building a solid foundation for your practice. Let's unpack these essential building blocks.

Understanding Mental Health Versus Mental Illness

Often, people use these terms interchangeably, but they represent different points on a spectrum. Think of it as a continuum, much like physical health.

Mental Health isn't simply the absence of illness. It's a state of **well-being**. It means you can generally:

- Realize your own abilities and potential.

- Cope with the normal stresses and strains of everyday life.

- Work productively and contribute to your community or family.

- Form positive relationships.

- Adapt to change and manage challenges.

Someone can have good mental health even while experiencing temporary sadness, grief, or stress—these are normal human responses. The key is the overall ability to function and find meaning in life. It's a dynamic state, fluctuating with life circumstances.

Mental Illness, on the other hand, refers to **diagnosable conditions** that affect a person's thinking, feeling, mood, or behavior. These conditions cause distress and/or impair functioning in social, occupational, or other significant areas of life. Examples include major depressive disorder, schizophrenia, bipolar disorder, panic disorder, and obsessive-compulsive disorder. These are medical conditions, just like diabetes or heart disease, often involving biological, psychological, and social factors.

The Continuum: It's crucial to see these not as absolute opposites but as points on a continuum.

- A person can have a diagnosed mental illness (like anxiety) but experience periods of good mental health and high functioning through effective management (medication, therapy, coping skills).

- Conversely, someone without a diagnosed mental illness might experience poor mental health due to overwhelming stress, grief, or difficult circumstances, leading to impaired functioning, even if temporary.

Why does this distinction matter for nurses?

Recognizing this continuum helps us avoid labeling people. We see the person first, not just the diagnosis. It allows us to focus on promoting well-being and resilience for all individuals, regardless of diagnosis, and to understand that functioning can vary greatly even among people with the same condition. It also helps combat stigma—mental illness isn't a personal failing; it's a health condition existing on a spectrum we are all on.

Case Study: The Health-Illness Continuum

- *Scenario:* Consider two colleagues, Anna and Ben, working in a high-pressure sales environment. Both face an unexpected corporate restructuring causing job uncertainty.

- *Anna:* Anna has no history of diagnosed mental illness. She feels stressed, has trouble sleeping for a week, and is irritable with her family. She talks with her partner, increases her exercise routine, and focuses on updating her resume. While experiencing poor mental health temporarily due to the stressor, she utilizes coping mechanisms and maintains overall functioning. She remains on the healthier end of the continuum, experiencing a normal reaction to stress.

- *Ben:* Ben has a history of generalized anxiety disorder, usually well-managed with medication and occasional therapy. The job stress significantly exacerbates his anxiety. He experiences panic attacks, constant worry, inability to concentrate at work, severe insomnia, and withdraws from social contact. His functioning is markedly impaired. He recognizes these signs as a worsening of his diagnosed condition. Ben is experiencing both a mental illness *and* poor mental health, requiring him to seek additional support from his therapist and possibly adjust his medication.

- *Nursing Perspective:* A nurse encountering Anna might offer stress management resources or employee assistance program information. For Ben, the nurse (perhaps an occupational health nurse or primary care nurse) would recognize the exacerbation of a known condition, assess the severity of symptoms (including safety), encourage him to follow up with his mental health providers, and reinforce coping strategies learned in therapy. Understanding the continuum allows the nurse to tailor the approach appropriately.

Key Theoretical Models Simplified Overview

How we understand and treat mental illness has changed over time, influenced by different ways of thinking—different models. No single model explains everything, but each offers a lens through which to view behavior and guide interventions. As nurses, having a basic grasp of these helps us understand *why* certain treatments are used and appreciate the multifaceted nature of mental health.

1. **Psychoanalytic Model (Freud and followers):**

   o **Core Idea:** Unconscious thoughts, desires, and conflicts, often rooted in early childhood experiences, drive behavior and can lead to psychological distress. Defense mechanisms (like denial or repression) are used to cope with anxiety arising from these conflicts.

   o **Simplified View:** Our past shapes our present, often in ways we aren't fully aware of. Problems arise from unresolved internal conflicts.

   o **Nursing Relevance:** While intensive psychoanalysis is done by specialists, this model highlights the importance of **listening for underlying themes**, understanding **past experiences** (like trauma) and their impact, recognizing **defense mechanisms** in patients, and the significance of the **therapeutic relationship** itself (transference/countertransference concepts originated here). It reminds us that behavior has meaning, even if it seems irrational at first glance.

24

2. **Behavioral Model (Pavlov, Skinner, Watson):**

   o **Core Idea:** Behaviors—both adaptive and maladaptive—are learned through interaction with the environment. Focus is on observable actions, not internal thoughts. Key concepts include classical conditioning (learning by association, like Pavlov's dogs), operant conditioning (learning through rewards and punishments), and modeling (learning by observing others).

   o **Simplified View:** We learn how to act based on experiences and consequences. What gets rewarded tends to be repeated.

   o **Nursing Relevance:** This model is the basis for many practical nursing interventions: **behavior modification plans** (rewarding desired behaviors), **token economies** on inpatient units, **exposure therapy** for phobias (gradually facing feared stimuli), **relaxation techniques**, and **skills training** (teaching coping skills, social skills). It emphasizes clear, measurable goals and tracking progress.

3. **Cognitive Model (Beck, Ellis):**

   o **Core Idea:** Thoughts, beliefs, and interpretations of events—not just the events themselves—cause emotional distress and maladaptive behavior. Faulty or distorted thinking patterns (e.g., "I'm worthless," "Everything always goes wrong") lead to negative feelings and actions.

   o **Simplified View:** How we *think* affects how we *feel* and *act*. Changing negative thoughts can change feelings and behaviors.

- **Nursing Relevance:** This is hugely influential in current practice. Nurses use cognitive principles when: **helping patients identify negative thought patterns** ("cognitive distortions"), **challenging unrealistic beliefs**, teaching **cognitive restructuring** (reframing thoughts), promoting **problem-solving skills**, and supporting Cognitive Behavioral Therapy (CBT). It empowers patients by showing them they can influence their feelings by changing their thinking.

4. **Biological Model (Medical Model):**

   - **Core Idea:** Mental illnesses are viewed as diseases with a biological basis, often involving genetics, brain structure abnormalities, or neurotransmitter imbalances (like serotonin, dopamine, norepinephrine).

   - **Simplified View:** Mental illness is caused by physical problems in the brain or body chemistry.

   - **Nursing Relevance:** This model underpins **psychopharmacology**. Understanding neurotransmitters helps explain how medications work. It guides **physical health assessment** (ruling out medical causes for psychiatric symptoms), **medication administration and monitoring**, educating patients about the biological aspects of their illness (which can reduce self-blame), and understanding **genetic predispositions**.

Putting Models Together: In practice, nurses rarely use just one model. We typically draw from all of them, recognizing that mental illness arises from a mixture of biological vulnerabilities, learned behaviors, thought patterns, past experiences, and

26

social factors. This integrated approach is often called the **Biopsychosocial Model**.

Case Study: Explaining Social Avoidance

- *Scenario:* Mark, a 30-year-old man, avoids social gatherings, calls in sick frequently, and has trouble maintaining friendships, despite expressing loneliness. How might different models view this?

  - *Psychoanalytic Lens:* Perhaps Mark had early childhood experiences of rejection or criticism, leading to an unconscious fear of judgment and defensive withdrawal.

  - *Behavioral Lens:* Maybe Mark had negative experiences at past social events (e.g., panic attack, being ridiculed) and learned to associate social situations with anxiety (classical conditioning). Avoiding them reduces anxiety, reinforcing the avoidance behavior (operant conditioning).

  - *Cognitive Lens:* Mark might hold core beliefs like "I'm awkward," or "People won't like me." He anticipates rejection, interprets neutral interactions negatively ("They were just being polite"), and focuses on his own perceived flaws during social events, increasing anxiety and confirming his negative beliefs.

  - *Biological Lens:* Mark might have a genetic predisposition to anxiety disorders, perhaps involving an overactive amygdala or imbalances in serotonin or GABA systems, making him more sensitive to social stress.

- *Nursing Approach:* An effective nursing approach would integrate these insights. The nurse might explore Mark's past experiences (Psychoanalytic), help him gradually face social situations with coping skills (Behavioral), challenge his negative thoughts and beliefs (Cognitive), and manage his anxiety symptoms, possibly supporting medication adherence if prescribed (Biological).

The Stress-Diathesis Model Explained

This is a highly useful framework for understanding how mental illness often develops. It bridges the gap between nature (biology/genetics) and nurture (environment/experiences).

- **Diathesis:** Refers to a **predisposition** or **vulnerability** to developing a disorder. This can be biological (e.g., genetic inheritance, brain structure differences), psychological (e.g., certain personality traits, early trauma), or sociocultural (e.g., growing up in poverty). Think of the diathesis as "loading the gun."

- **Stress:** Refers to **environmental or life stressors** that trigger the onset of the disorder in someone with a diathesis. Stressors can be biological (e.g., substance use, infection), psychological (e.g., loss of a loved one, job loss, relationship problems), or social (e.g., discrimination, abuse, major life changes). Think of stress as "pulling the trigger."

The Core Idea: Neither the diathesis nor the stress alone is usually enough to cause the disorder. It's the **combination**—the interaction between the predisposition and the triggering stress—that leads to the development of mental illness.

- Someone with a **strong diathesis** (e.g., strong family history of schizophrenia) might develop the illness even with relatively mild stressors.

- Someone with a **weaker diathesis** might only develop the illness under conditions of extreme or prolonged stress.

- Some individuals with a diathesis may never encounter sufficient stress to trigger the illness and remain healthy.

Analogy: Imagine two people inherit genes making them susceptible to depression (diathesis). Both lose their jobs (stress). Person A, with strong social support and coping skills (protective factors), experiences sadness but recovers. Person B, who lacks support and has past trauma, develops Major Depressive Disorder. The same stressor had different outcomes due to differing vulnerabilities and protective factors.

Nursing Relevance:

- Helps explain why some people develop illness under stress while others don't.

- Guides assessment—we need to ask about both **family history/vulnerabilities** (diathesis) and **recent life events/stressors**.

- Highlights the importance of **stress management** and **coping skills** (reducing the impact of stressors).

- Emphasizes building **protective factors** (like social support, resilience) to buffer against stress.

- Provides a hopeful framework—even with a diathesis, illness isn't inevitable if stress can be managed or protective factors strengthened.

Recovery Model Principles

The Recovery Model represents a significant shift in thinking about mental health care, moving away from a sole focus on eliminating symptoms (like the traditional medical model) towards empowering individuals to live meaningful lives *chosen by them*, even if symptoms persist. It's a message of **hope and empowerment**.

Key principles include:

1. **Hope:** Believing recovery is possible is the foundation. Nurses instill hope by sharing stories of success (appropriately), celebrating small steps, and focusing on strengths.

2. **Person-Driven:** Individuals define their own life goals and direct their own care. Planning is collaborative ("doing *with*," not "doing *to*"). Nurses support self-determination and informed choices.

3. **Many Pathways:** Recovery is non-linear and unique to each person. Setbacks are part of the process, not failures. Nurses support individuals through ups and downs, respecting diverse paths (therapy, medication, peer support, lifestyle changes, spirituality, etc.).

4. **Holistic:** Recovery involves the whole person—mind, body, spirit, community. It addresses trauma, promotes wellness (housing, employment, education), and integrates physical and mental health care.

5. **Peer Support:** Individuals with lived experience offer invaluable support, encouragement, and hope. Nurses connect patients with peer specialists and support groups.

6. **Relational:** Positive relationships (family, friends, providers) are crucial. Nurses build trusting, respectful relationships.

7. **Culture:** Culture shapes experiences and recovery paths. Services should be culturally sensitive and relevant. (More on this next).

8. **Addresses Trauma:** Recognizing the prevalence of trauma and providing trauma-informed care is essential.

9. **Strengths/Responsibility:** Focus on individual strengths, coping abilities, and resources. Support individuals in taking responsibility for their recovery journey.

10. **Respect:** Protecting rights, eliminating discrimination, and promoting social inclusion are fundamental.

Recovery vs. Cure: Recovery doesn't necessarily mean cure or the complete absence of illness. It means living a satisfying, hopeful life despite limitations caused by illness.

Nursing Relevance:

The Recovery Model profoundly impacts nursing practice:

- Shifts focus from just symptom management to **promoting quality of life, goals, and functioning.**

- Requires **collaborative goal setting** and care planning with the patient.

- Emphasizes **strengths-based assessment**—what *can* the person do? What are their resources?

- Promotes **patient education and empowerment** to manage their own condition.

- Encourages connection with **peer support** and community resources.

- Requires **hopeful and respectful communication.**

Case Study: Recovery in Action

- *Scenario:* Lisa, diagnosed with Bipolar I Disorder, has frequent hospitalizations during manic episodes. A traditional approach focused solely on medication adherence and preventing relapse. Using a Recovery Model approach, her nurse, Chen, works differently.

- *Nurse's Action (Recovery-Oriented):* Chen asks Lisa about her *life goals*, not just symptom control. Lisa tearfully shares her dream of finishing her art degree, abandoned years ago due to illness instability. Together, they create a plan:

    o *Goal:* Re-enroll in one art class next semester.

    o *Steps:*

        ▪ Maintain medication adherence (biological).

        ▪ Develop a structured daily routine to manage mood swings (behavioral/cognitive).

        ▪ Identify early warning signs of mania/depression and create a 'wellness plan' for responding (cognitive/self-management).

        ▪ Connect with the university's disability services for potential accommodations (strengths/resources).

        ▪ Join a bipolar support group for peer connection (relational/peer support).

        ▪ Explore stress management techniques like mindfulness (holistic).

- *Outcome:* Lisa experiences setbacks, including a mild hypomanic episode where she wants to enroll in five classes. Chen helps her revisit the plan, acknowledge her ambition (strength), but gently guide her back to the agreed-upon single class to avoid overwhelming stress (person-driven but responsible). Over time, Lisa successfully completes classes, builds confidence, and feels her life has purpose beyond just managing her illness. She defines her recovery not by the absence of bipolar disorder, but by her ability to pursue her goals and live well *with* it.

Cultural Considerations in Mental Health

Culture—the shared beliefs, values, customs, language, and practices of a group—profoundly influences how people understand, express, and cope with mental health issues. What's considered "normal" behavior in one culture might be seen as pathological in another. Ignoring cultural context can lead to misdiagnosis, ineffective treatment, and mistrust.

Key considerations for nurses:

- **Expression of Distress:** Symptoms manifest differently. Someone from a culture emphasizing stoicism might express depression through physical complaints (somatization) rather than verbalizing sadness. Someone from another culture might express distress through spiritual or religious idioms.

- **Beliefs about Causation:** Cultures have varying beliefs about what causes mental illness (e.g., spiritual imbalance, witchcraft, genetics, life stress). Understanding this helps frame discussions about treatment.

- **Stigma Levels:** While stigma exists globally, its intensity and focus vary. In some cultures, mental illness brings great shame to the entire family.

- **Help-Seeking Behaviors:** Who do people turn to first? Family? Elders? Religious leaders? Traditional healers? Doctors? Understanding preferred pathways is key.

- **Family Dynamics:** The role of the family varies greatly. In collectivist cultures, family involvement in decision-making may be expected and necessary.

- **Treatment Preferences:** Preferences for medication versus therapy, traditional healing practices, or spiritual interventions differ.

- **Communication Styles:** Norms around eye contact, personal space, emotional expression, and directness vary. Language barriers are also a major factor.

Cultural Humility vs. Cultural Competence:

- **Cultural Competence** suggests one can *master* knowledge about other cultures. This is often unrealistic given the diversity within any group.

- **Cultural Humility** is a preferred approach. It involves:

    o A lifelong commitment to **self-evaluation and self-critique**.

    o Recognizing and challenging **power imbalances** in the[16] patient-provider relationship.

    o Developing **partnerships** with communities.

    o Holding institutions **accountable**.

    o Most importantly: Approaching each person as an individual, asking them about *their* beliefs and preferences, rather than assuming based on their cultural background. **"Ask, don't assume."**

Nursing Implications:

- **Self-Reflection:** Examine your own cultural biases.

- **Assessment:** Ask about cultural background, beliefs about illness/treatment, important values, family roles, and language preferences. Use trained interpreters when needed—never family members for complex issues.

- **Communication:** Adapt your style respectfully. Be mindful of nonverbal cues.

- **Treatment Planning:** Incorporate patient/family beliefs and preferences whenever possible and safe. Collaborate with traditional healers if appropriate and desired by the patient.

- **Advocacy:** Advocate for culturally appropriate services and resources.

Case Study: Cultural Sensitivity

- *Scenario:* Mr. Lee, a 70-year-old recent immigrant from rural China, is brought to the clinic by his son. He reports vague physical complaints (fatigue, aches) but denies feeling sad or depressed. His son explains that Mr. Lee hasn't left the house much since his wife died six months ago and seems to have lost interest in everything. The GP suspects depression.

- *Nurse's Action (Culturally Humble):* The nurse, Maria, avoids immediately labeling Mr. Lee as depressed based on Western criteria. She uses a trained interpreter.

    o She asks Mr. Lee to describe his symptoms *in his own words*. He focuses on physical discomfort and "imbalance."

    o She asks about his understanding of his symptoms – "What do you think might be causing these feelings?" He mentions grief and disharmony.

- She asks about coping – "What usually helps you feel better when you are unwell or grieving?" He mentions certain herbal teas and spending time with family.

- She asks about family involvement – "How does your family usually support each other during difficult times?" The son explains the importance of family presence and respect for elders.

- Maria explains depression using neutral terms, linking it to imbalance and stress, possibly validating his physical symptoms as part of the picture. She discusses treatment options, including medication (explaining potential benefits simply) and counseling (explaining it as talking through worries), but also asks if incorporating traditional practices like tea or involving family more would be helpful.

- *Outcome:* Mr. Lee feels respected. He agrees to try medication, reassured it might help restore balance, but emphasizes the importance of family visits. The son feels included. The care plan incorporates both Western medicine and culturally meaningful support, increasing the likelihood of engagement and effectiveness. Maria avoided imposing her cultural framework and instead collaborated based on Mr. Lee's perspective.

Key Term Quick Reference

- **Mental Health:** State of well-being enabling coping, productivity, contribution, and realizing potential.

- **Mental Illness:** Diagnosable condition affecting thoughts/feelings/behavior, causing distress or functional impairment.

- **Continuum:** Concept that mental health and illness exist on a spectrum, not as absolutes.

- **Theoretical Model:** A framework or way of thinking used to explain phenomena (e.g., behavior, illness). Examples: Psychoanalytic, Behavioral, Cognitive, Biological.

- **Biopsychosocial Model:** Integrated approach viewing illness as arising from biological, psychological, and social factors.

- **Diathesis:** Predisposition or vulnerability (biological/psychological/social).

- **Stress (Stress-Diathesis Model):** Environmental or life events that trigger illness in vulnerable individuals.

- **Recovery Model:** Philosophy emphasizing hope, self-determination, holistic care, strengths, and living meaningfully despite illness.

- **Culture:** Shared beliefs, values, practices of a group influencing health behaviors and understanding.

- **Cultural Humility:** Lifelong process of self-reflection and learning, approaching others with humility and respect for their individual cultural perspective.

- **Stigma:** Negative attitudes, beliefs, and discrimination towards people with mental health conditions.

- **Person-First Language:** Describing the person before the diagnosis (e.g., "person with depression").

(Concept Map Idea: A central circle labeled "Mental Health Condition" with arrows pointing to it from surrounding circles

labeled "Biological Factors (Genetics, Neurotransmitters),"
"Psychological Factors (Trauma, Thoughts, Coping)," and
"Social/Cultural Factors (Stress, Support, Stigma)." Arrows could
also show interplay between the factors. Another simple map
could show "Diathesis (Vulnerability)" + "Stressors" leading to
"Potential for Illness," buffered by "Protective Factors.")

A Thought on Frameworks

These concepts and models aren't just abstract ideas; they are
the lenses through which we view the people we care for.
Understanding the difference between health and illness helps
us see potential. Knowing the theoretical models gives us
multiple ways to understand behavior. Appreciating the
interplay of stress and vulnerability guides our assessments.
Embracing recovery principles fosters hope. And recognizing
cultural influences ensures respectful, individualized care. They
provide a map—not dictating the journey, but helping us
navigate the work ahead with greater understanding and
purpose. Now, let's turn to the cornerstone of putting this
understanding into practice: the therapeutic relationship.

Core Learnings from This Section

- Mental health and illness exist on a **continuum**; focus on
  promoting well-being for all.

- Major theoretical models (**Psychoanalytic, Behavioral,
  Cognitive, Biological**) offer different perspectives on
  mental illness; an integrated **Biopsychosocial** approach
  is often best.

- The **Stress-Diathesis Model** explains how vulnerability
  interacts with stressors to trigger illness.

- The **Recovery Model** emphasizes **hope, person-driven goals, strengths, and living meaningfully**, shifting focus from mere symptom control.

- **Culture** significantly impacts the expression, understanding, and treatment of mental health; practice **cultural humility** by asking, not assuming.

- These foundational concepts directly inform nursing assessment, intervention, and communication.

Chapter 2: The Therapeutic Relationship Tool

In mental health nursing, perhaps more than any other specialty, the **relationship** between the nurse and the patient is not just *part* of the treatment—it *is* a primary therapeutic tool. It's within the context of a trusting, respectful connection that assessment becomes accurate, interventions become effective, and healing can begin. Think of it as the operating table or the sterile field of psychiatric care; without it, our other tools lose much of their power. Building and maintaining this relationship requires specific skills, conscious effort, and unwavering professional integrity.

Building Trust and Rapport

Trust isn't automatic; it's earned. Many individuals seeking mental health care have experienced broken trust or difficult relationships in the past. They may be wary, skeptical, or frightened. Building rapport—a sense of connection and mutual understanding—is the first step.

How do you build trust and rapport?

1. **Consistency:** Do what you say you will do. If you promise to return at a certain time, return at that time. If you schedule time to talk, keep that appointment. Predictability builds security.

2. **Honesty and Authenticity:** Be truthful (within professional boundaries). Don't make promises you can't keep. Be genuine in your interactions—patients can often sense insincerity. If you don't know an answer, say so, and offer to find out.

3. **Respect and Non-Judgment:** View the patient as a person worthy of dignity, regardless of their diagnosis, behavior, or background. Listen without judgment. Use

person-first language. Respect their opinions and choices, even if you don't agree with them.

4. **Empathy:** Strive to understand the patient's world from *their* perspective. Communicate that understanding back to them. (We'll discuss empathy vs. sympathy more soon).

5. **Active Listening:** Pay full attention when the patient is speaking. Show you are listening through nonverbal cues (nodding, eye contact as appropriate) and verbal cues (reflecting, clarifying). Make them feel heard.

6. **Confidentiality:** Clearly explain the limits of confidentiality (harm to self/others, abuse) upfront. Assure them that within those limits, what they share is private. Uphold that promise rigorously.

7. **Providing Clear Information:** Explain procedures, medications, and the plan of care in understandable language. Uncertainty breeds anxiety; clarity builds trust.

8. **Patience:** Trust takes time, especially with individuals who are guarded or have experienced trauma. Don't rush the process. Allow the relationship to develop at the patient's pace.

Case Study: Earning Trust Through Consistency

- *Scenario:* Mr. Peters, a 45-year-old man with chronic schizophrenia and a history of treatment non-adherence, is admitted to the inpatient unit after neglecting his self-care and experiencing increased paranoia. He is withdrawn, suspicious, speaks little, and avoids eye contact. He refuses group activities and often stays in his room.

- *Nurse's Action:* Sarah, his primary nurse, understands that building trust will be slow.

    o *Day 1:* Sarah introduces herself calmly, explains her role simply, and tells Mr. Peters she will check on him briefly every hour during her shift. She keeps her interactions short and non-demanding initially. She arrives promptly each hour, even if just to say hello briefly at his doorway if he seems unreceptive.

    o *Day 2:* She continues the consistent checks. She brings him his medication, explaining what it is and its purpose clearly, without pressure. When he refuses, she calmly acknowledges his refusal, documents it, and informs the treatment team, stating she will offer it again later. She notices he hasn't eaten much and asks, "Mr. Peters, I see you haven't touched your lunch. Is there something specific you might prefer?" (He shrugs).

    o *Day 3:* During her hourly check, Sarah finds Mr. Peters sitting on his bed. She says, "Mr. Peters, I have about 10 minutes before my next task. I could spend it here with you, if you like. We don't have to talk." He gives a slight nod. Sarah pulls up a chair and sits quietly nearby. After several minutes of silence, he quietly says, "They watch me." Sarah replies calmly, using reflection, "You feel like you are being watched?" He nods.

    o *Ongoing:* Sarah continues her consistent, predictable, non-judgmental approach. She offers medication regularly, respects his refusals while gently re-offering, spends brief, scheduled time with him (gradually increasing as tolerated), and focuses on meeting basic needs (food, hygiene) without demands.

- *Outcome:* Over several days, Mr. Peters begins to make brief eye contact. He starts accepting his medication occasionally. He answers Sarah's questions with more than one word. While still guarded, his willingness to engage slightly demonstrates a nascent trust built on Sarah's reliability, respect for his space, and non-pressuring presence. This foundation is essential before deeper therapeutic work can occur.

Professional Boundaries Do's and Don'ts

Professional boundaries are the limits that protect the space between the nurse's professional power and the patient's vulnerability. They keep the relationship **safe, therapeutic, and focused on the patient's needs**. Maintaining boundaries isn't about being cold or distant; it's about ensuring professionalism and ethical integrity.

Why are boundaries so important in mental health?

- **Patient Vulnerability:** Patients are often emotionally vulnerable and may have difficulty with relationships.

- **Nurse's Power:** The nurse inherently holds a position of power (access to information, institutional authority).

- **Transference/Countertransference:** Patients may unconsciously transfer feelings from past relationships onto the nurse (transference). Nurses may unconsciously transfer feelings onto the patient (countertransference). Boundaries help manage these phenomena.

- **Risk of Exploitation:** Clear boundaries prevent exploitation, even unintentional.

Key Boundary Considerations: Do's

- **Do** maintain confidentiality strictly (within legal limits).

- **Do** provide care equitably to all patients, regardless of personal feelings.

- **Do** use therapeutic communication techniques.

- **Do** focus interactions on the patient's needs and goals.

- **Do** dress and act professionally.

- **Do** be mindful of the length and time of sessions/interactions.

- **Do** document interactions objectively.

- **Do** consult with colleagues or supervisors if you feel boundary issues arising.

Key Boundary Considerations: Don'ts

- **Don't** engage in social relationships with patients (during or after treatment). No dating, no becoming "friends" on social media.

- **Don't** accept significant gifts, loans, or tips from patients (check institutional policy on small tokens).

- **Don't** give patients personal contact information (phone number, email, address).

- **Don't** engage in extensive self-disclosure about your personal life, problems, or strong opinions. Keep the focus on the patient. (Limited, purposeful self-disclosure can *sometimes* be therapeutic, but requires careful judgment and supervision).

- **Don't** perform special favors for one patient that you wouldn't do for others.

- **Don't** keep secrets with patients from the rest of the treatment team.

- **Don't** engage in physical contact beyond what's professionally appropriate and necessary for care (e.g., avoid casual hugging unless culturally appropriate and clearly welcomed *by the patient*).

- **Don't** make promises you cannot keep.

Boundary Crossings vs. Boundary Violations:

- **Boundary Crossing:** A brief, often unintentional, step over the line. It might be accepting a small handmade card, or briefly self-disclosing something relevant. Crossings *can sometimes* be therapeutic if done thoughtfully, but they warrant careful examination. They are generally benign and non-exploitative.

- **Boundary Violation:** A more serious breach that is potentially or actually harmful or exploitative. Examples include engaging in a romantic relationship, accepting large sums of money, keeping harmful secrets, or exploiting the patient's vulnerability for personal gain. Violations are *always* unprofessional and unethical.

Red Flags for Boundary Problems (in the Nurse):

- Thinking about the patient frequently outside of work.

- Spending disproportionately more time with one patient.

- Feeling you are the *only* one who understands the patient.

- Sharing detailed personal problems with the patient.

- Keeping secrets with the patient.

- Feeling defensive when colleagues ask about your relationship with the patient.

- Receiving or giving gifts.

- Engaging in social contact outside of treatment.

If you notice these signs in yourself or a colleague, it's essential to seek supervision or consultation immediately.

Case Study: Navigating a Boundary Challenge

- *Scenario:* Clara, a young woman admitted for depression, forms a strong rapport with her nurse, David. She starts sharing details about her difficult relationship with her boyfriend, similar to problems David experienced years ago. Clara tells David, "You're the only one who really gets it. Can I call you after I leave here if I need someone to talk to?" She also brings him a small, inexpensive keychain she bought from the hospital gift shop.

- *David's Actions (Maintaining Boundaries):*

  - *Regarding the Phone Call:* David recognizes Clara's feeling of connection but knows providing his number is inappropriate. He responds kindly but firmly: "Clara, I really appreciate you feeling comfortable talking with me, and I'm glad we've been able to work together here. However, my role as your nurse is while you're in the hospital. It wouldn't be professional for me to have contact outside of that. Let's make sure we develop a really strong discharge plan with resources you *can* call, like a therapist or a helpline, for ongoing support." (Focuses on patient needs, clarifies role, offers appropriate alternatives).

  - *Regarding Self-Disclosure:* David feels tempted to share his own past relationship issues to show understanding but resists. He realizes this would shift the focus away from Clara and blur the professional line. Instead, he uses empathy: "It sounds like that relationship causes you a lot of pain and frustration." (Keeps focus on Clara's feelings).

- o *Regarding the Gift:* David checks his hospital's policy. Small, inexpensive tokens are generally acceptable. He accepts the keychain graciously: "Thank you, Clara, that's thoughtful of you." He avoids making a big deal of it and doesn't offer a gift in return. (Follows policy, maintains professionalism).

- *Outcome:* David successfully navigates potential boundary issues. He validates Clara's feelings and trust in him but maintains professional limits regarding contact and self-disclosure, ensuring the relationship remains therapeutic and focused on her discharge planning and long-term support needs. He handles the small gift according to policy, preserving the rapport without compromising boundaries.

Empathy Versus Sympathy

These terms are often confused, but the difference is critical in therapeutic relationships.

- **Empathy: The ability to understand and share the feelings of another person from *their* frame of reference**. It's putting yourself in their shoes and seeing the world (or the situation) as they see it, even if you don't feel the same way yourself. It involves cognitive understanding ("I understand why you feel that way") and affective connection ("I sense how difficult that must be for you"). Empathy communicates understanding and validation.

47

○ *Example:* Patient says, "I feel like such a failure."
Empathetic response: "It sounds like you're
feeling really down on yourself right now, like
things haven't worked out as you hoped."
(Reflects understanding of the feeling).

- **Sympathy: Feeling pity or sorrow for someone else's
misfortune**. It's feeling *for* the person, rather than *with*
them. While well-intentioned, sympathy often creates
distance. It focuses on your own feelings ("I feel so sorry
for you") rather than the patient's experience. It can
sometimes come across as patronizing or minimize the
person's strength.

○ *Example:* Patient says, "I feel like such a failure."
Sympathetic response: "Oh, you poor thing,
that's terrible! Don't feel that way." (Focuses on
pity, offers platitude).

Why is Empathy Therapeutic?

- **Builds Trust:** Feeling understood fosters connection.

- **Validates Feelings:** It communicates that the patient's
feelings are real and understandable in their context.

- **Encourages Exploration:** When patients feel understood,
they are more likely to explore their feelings and
experiences further.

- **Reduces Alienation:** It helps patients feel less alone in
their struggles.

- **Empowers:** By understanding their perspective, you can
better help them find their *own* solutions.

Why Can Sympathy Be Less Helpful (or even harmful)?

- **Creates Distance:** It highlights the difference between
the "helper" and the "helped."

- **Can Feel Patronizing:** Pity can make people feel diminished.

- **May Discourage Problem-Solving:** Focusing on feeling sorry might overshadow exploring solutions.

- **Focuses on the Nurse's Feelings:** Shifts the focus away from the patient.

Developing Empathy:

Empathy isn't just about feeling; it's a skill that can be developed:

- **Practice Active Listening:** Really hear what the patient is saying, verbally and nonverbally.

- **Be Self-Aware:** Recognize your own biases and feelings so they don't interfere with understanding the patient.

- **Seek Understanding:** Ask clarifying questions to grasp their perspective ("Can you tell me more about what that was like for you?").

- **Communicate Understanding:** Use reflective statements ("It sounds like...", "You seem to be feeling...", "So, for you, it was like...").

Empathy is the engine of the therapeutic relationship—it allows you to connect meaningfully and effectively support the patient's journey.

Phases of the Nurse Client Relationship Simplified Peplau

Hildegard Peplau, a pioneering nursing theorist, described the nurse-patient relationship as developing in overlapping phases. Understanding these phases helps nurses anticipate and navigate the dynamics of the relationship effectively. Here's a simplified look:

1. **Orientation (or Introductory) Phase:**

- **Goal:** Establish trust, define roles, identify patient needs/problems, agree on a preliminary plan or "contract" for working together.

- **Nurse's Role:** Introduce self, explain role/purpose, set boundaries (confidentiality, time limits), listen actively, build rapport, gather assessment data, help patient identify problems.

- **Patient's Behavior:** May be anxious, hesitant, testing the nurse's reliability and sincerity, asking questions, trying to understand rules and expectations.

- **Key Task:** Building a foundation of trust and defining the work to be done.

2. **Working Phase:**

- **Goal:** Explore problems in depth, promote insight, develop coping skills, facilitate behavior change, evaluate progress. This is where most of the therapeutic work happens.

- **Nurse's Role:** Use therapeutic communication techniques (reflecting, focusing, confronting gently), help patient explore thoughts/feelings/behaviors, implement care plan interventions (education, skills training), provide feedback, support patient in trying new behaviors, manage challenging dynamics like transference (patient projects past feelings onto nurse) and countertransference (nurse projects feelings onto patient – requires supervision!).

- **Patient's Behavior:** Actively participates (ideally), explores issues, experiences strong emotions, tests boundaries again, may show resistance or ambivalence about change, practices new skills, develops insight.

- o **Key Task:** Addressing the patient's issues and facilitating change.

3. **Termination (or Resolution) Phase:**

- o **Goal:** Review progress made, prepare for the end of the relationship (e.g., discharge, transfer), manage feelings associated with ending, plan for future needs and relapse prevention.

- o **Nurse's Role:** Initiate discussion about termination well in advance, encourage patient to reflect on progress and experience, validate feelings about ending (sadness, anger, anxiety), summarize work done, reinforce coping strategies, discuss follow-up plans and resources.

- o **Patient's Behavior:** May express sadness or anxiety about ending, minimize progress or regress temporarily, test boundaries one last time, share feelings about the relationship, participate in planning for the future.

- o **Key Task:** Bringing closure to the relationship constructively and preparing the patient for independence.

Important Notes:

- These phases are **overlapping**, not strictly sequential. You might revisit orientation phase issues during the working phase.

- The **length** of each phase varies greatly depending on the setting (acute care vs. long-term therapy) and the patient's needs.

- Being aware of the **tasks and potential dynamics** of each phase helps the nurse anticipate challenges and respond therapeutically.

Case Study: Moving Through the Phases

- *Scenario:* A nurse, Maria, works with Alex, a young adult admitted for severe anxiety and social phobia, over several weeks on an inpatient unit preparing for a partial hospitalization program.

    - *Orientation:* In the first few sessions, Maria focuses on building trust. Alex is quiet, anxious, avoids eye contact. Maria explains her role, meeting times, and confidentiality. She asks open-ended questions about what brought Alex to the hospital. Alex tests her by being late for one session. Maria addresses it gently ("Alex, we agreed to meet at 10. It's important we stick to our time to make the most of it."). They identify initial goals: attending group therapy and managing panic symptoms.

    - *Working:* Over the next weeks, Maria uses active listening and reflection as Alex shares fears of judgment. They explore negative thought patterns contributing to anxiety (cognitive). Maria teaches relaxation and grounding techniques (behavioral). Alex practices these skills, sometimes successfully, sometimes struggling. He expresses frustration. Maria validates the difficulty but encourages persistence. They discuss his anxieties about the upcoming partial hospitalization program. Maria recognizes Alex sometimes seems overly dependent on her approval (possible transference) and discusses this pattern gently, linking it to his fear of judgment.

- o *Termination:* A week before discharge to the partial program, Maria reminds Alex their sessions will be ending. Alex becomes withdrawn again, saying, "I don't think I'm ready." Maria explores his feelings ("It sounds scary to leave the unit"), reviews the coping skills he learned, summarizes his progress (attending groups, reduced panic attacks), and frames the partial program as the next step in his recovery journey, not an abandonment. They finalize his follow-up plan and resource list. On the last day, Alex thanks Maria, stating he feels nervous but more prepared.

- *Outcome:* By understanding the phases, Maria guides the relationship purposefully—building trust initially, actively working on goals, and preparing Alex for a smooth transition by addressing termination appropriately.

Communication Tips Quick Reference

- **Be Consistent:** Predictability builds trust.

- **Listen More, Talk Less:** Let the patient lead.

- **Use Open-Ended Questions:** "Tell me more...", "How did that feel?"

- **Reflect Feelings:** "It sounds like you're feeling..."

- **Validate Concerns:** "I can understand why you might feel that way."

- **Be Honest & Clear:** Avoid jargon and false promises.

- **Maintain Professional Boundaries:** Keep the focus on the patient's needs.

- **Silence Can Be Therapeutic:** Allow time for reflection.

Boundary Violation Red Flags

- Excessive self-disclosure by the nurse.

- Secret-keeping with the patient.

- Social contact outside of therapy/care setting.

- Accepting or giving significant gifts.

- Feeling possessive or that you're the "only one" who helps.

- Spending disproportionate time with one patient.

- Dressing differently for a specific patient.

- Strong emotional reactions (positive or negative) to a patient (seek supervision!).

A Thought on Connection

The therapeutic relationship is where the science of nursing meets the art of human connection. It demands technical skill— knowing *how* to listen, *when* to speak, *what* boundaries to hold. But it also requires those inherently human qualities of warmth, genuineness, and the capacity to truly see and hear another person without judgment. It is within this carefully constructed, ethically sound, and empathetically engaged space that patients find the safety to confront their struggles and discover their strengths. Master this, and you master the heart of mental health nursing. Next, we will look more closely at the specific techniques that bring this relationship to life: therapeutic communication.

Core Learnings from This Section

- The **therapeutic nurse-patient relationship** is a primary tool in mental health care.

- **Trust and rapport** are foundational and built through consistency, honesty, respect, empathy, and active listening.

- **Professional boundaries** are essential for safety and effectiveness; know the Do's and Don'ts and recognize red flags for violations.

- **Empathy** (understanding from the patient's view) is therapeutic, while **sympathy** (feeling sorry for) can create distance.

- The relationship typically progresses through **Orientation, Working, and Termination phases** (Peplau), each with specific tasks and dynamics.

- Maintaining this relationship requires skill, self-awareness, and ethical integrity.

Chapter 3: Therapeutic Communication in Action

If the therapeutic relationship is the container for healing, then **therapeutic communication** is the active ingredient—the process through which connection is made, understanding is deepened, and change is facilitated. It's more than just talking; it's a purposeful, planned interaction aimed at meeting the patient's psychosocial needs. This requires specific skills and techniques, as well as an awareness of common pitfalls that can shut down communication. Let's look at how to communicate effectively.

Active Listening Techniques

You cannot communicate therapeutically if you are not truly listening. Active listening is about fully concentrating on what the patient is saying—and what they're *not* saying—understanding their message, and communicating that understanding back to them. It's far more than just remaining silent while someone else talks.

Components of Active Listening:

1. **Being Present:** Mentally and physically focused on the patient. Minimize distractions (internal thoughts, external noise). Put away your phone. Sit facing the patient (if culturally appropriate) with open body language.

2. **Observing Nonverbal Cues:** Pay attention to posture, facial expressions, eye contact (or lack thereof), tone of voice, gestures, and motor activity. Nonverbal communication often conveys more than words. Does their body language match their words?

3. **Listening for Themes and Patterns:** What are the recurring topics, feelings, or concerns the patient expresses? What underlying message might be present?

4. **Providing Verbal and Nonverbal Feedback:** Show you are engaged through:

   o **Nonverbal:** Nodding, leaning slightly forward, maintaining appropriate eye contact.

   o **Verbal:** Using brief encouragers ("Uh-huh," "Go on"), reflecting ("It sounds like you felt angry"), asking clarifying questions, paraphrasing ("So, if I understand correctly, you're saying..."), and summarizing.

5. **Listening Without Judgment:** Avoid interrupting with your own opinions, advice, or interpretations. Your goal is to understand *their* world, not impose yours.

Why is Active Listening so Foundational?

- Builds rapport and trust.

- Helps the patient feel heard and validated.

- Allows the nurse to gather accurate assessment data.

- Encourages the patient to explore their thoughts and feelings more deeply.

- Reduces the chance of misunderstandings.

Case Study: The Power of Being Heard

- *Scenario:* Ms. Evans, a 50-year-old woman admitted for anxiety, paces the hallway, wringing her hands. She approaches the nurse, Leo, and says quickly, "I can't stay here, I have too much to do at home, the kids need me, my boss will be furious, I just have to leave."

- *Leo's Action (Active Listening):* Instead of immediately arguing or trying to reassure her, Leo stops what he's doing, turns to face Ms. Evans, and uses active listening.

- o *(Being Present/Nonverbal):* He makes eye contact, maintains a calm expression, and nods slightly as she speaks.

- o *(Reflecting/Paraphrasing):* "It sounds like you're feeling overwhelmed with worries about responsibilities outside the hospital right now, Ms. Evans."

- o *(Observing Nonverbal):* He notes her pacing, hand-wringing, and rapid speech, recognizing signs of high anxiety.

- o *(Open-Ended Question):* "Tell me more about the things that are worrying you most right now."

- *Outcome:* Ms. Evans pauses her pacing. Validated, she begins to list her specific worries—an upcoming deadline, a child's school event. As she talks, her breathing slows slightly. By truly listening and reflecting her concerns, Leo helps her feel understood, which slightly de-escalates her anxiety and opens the door for problem-solving or teaching coping skills, rather than escalating into a power struggle about leaving.

Asking Effective Questions

The questions we ask can either open doors to understanding or shut them down. Therapeutic questioning aims to facilitate exploration, gather information, and promote insight—not interrogate.

Types of Questions:

1. **Open-Ended Questions:**

   - o **Purpose:** Encourage detailed responses, explore feelings and perceptions, allow the patient to lead the conversation.

- Format: Typically start with "What," "How," "Tell me about," "Could you describe..."

- Examples: "What has been troubling you lately?" "How did you feel when that happened?" "Tell me more about your relationship with your family." "Could you describe a typical day for you?"

- Use: Excellent for starting conversations, exploring broad topics, and understanding the patient's perspective.

2. **Closed-Ended Questions:**

  - **Purpose:** Elicit specific information, obtain facts, limit responses (often to "yes" or "no" or a short answer).

  - **Format:** Often start with "Are," "Do," "Did," "Is," "Will."

  - **Examples:** "Are you feeling suicidal right now?" "Did you take your medication this morning?" "Is your pain better or worse?" "Will you attend group today?"

  - **Use:** Necessary for specific assessments (like risk assessment, medication compliance), gathering factual data quickly, or refocusing a rambling conversation. Use sparingly when exploration is the goal.

3. **Clarifying Questions:**

  - **Purpose:** Ensure understanding when the patient's message is unclear, vague, or ambiguous.

- Format: "I'm not sure I understand...", "Could you explain that again?", "What do you mean by...?", "Can you give me an example?"

- Examples: "You said you feel 'stuck.' What does 'stuck' mean to you?" "I'm not sure I follow your train of thought. Could you go over that last part again?" "Give me an example of a time you felt that way."

- Use: Essential to prevent assumptions and ensure you accurately grasp the patient's meaning.

Effective Questioning Tips:

- **Use "What" or "How" more than "Why":** "Why" questions can sound accusatory and put people on the defensive (e.g., "Why did you stop taking your medication?"). Instead, try "What were some of the difficulties you had with the medication?" or "How did you decide to stop taking it?"

- **Ask one question at a time.** Avoid bombarding the patient.

- **Allow silence for reflection.** Don't rush to fill the space after asking a question.

- **Phrase questions neutrally.** Avoid leading questions that suggest a desired answer.

Therapeutic Techniques Versus Non Therapeutic Blocks

Nurses use specific verbal techniques to encourage patients to express feelings, develop insight, and consider change. Just as important is recognizing communication patterns that *block* therapeutic progress.

Common Therapeutic Techniques:

- **Offering Self:** Making oneself available without demanding interaction. "I'll sit with you for a while." "I'm available to talk if you'd like." (Shows presence and caring).

- **Using Silence:** Allowing pauses for reflection for both nurse and patient. Can convey acceptance and allow the patient to gather thoughts. (Requires nurse comfort with silence).

- **Making Observations:** Stating observed behaviors neutrally. "You seem tense today." "I notice you haven't eaten breakfast." (Encourages patient to recognize behavior and comment).

- **Reflecting:** Directing the patient's feelings, ideas, or questions back to them to encourage exploration. Patient: "Do you think I should...?" Nurse: "What do *you* think you should do?" Patient: "I feel so angry!" Nurse: "You feel angry." (Validates and encourages elaboration).

- **Restating (Paraphrasing):** Repeating the main idea the patient expressed in similar words. "So, you're saying that you felt frustrated when..." (Confirms understanding, encourages continuation).

- **Seeking Clarification:** Asking for more explanation when something is unclear. "Could you tell me more about that feeling?" "I'm not sure I understand what you mean by 'giving up'." (Ensures accurate understanding).

- **Focusing:** Concentrating attention on a single important point or feeling, especially if the patient is vague or rambling. "Let's go back to what you said about feeling afraid." "Of all the things you've mentioned, what is bothering you most right now?" (Helps organize thinking).

- **Presenting Reality:** Gently describing reality for a patient misinterpreting it (use cautiously, especially with firm delusions). "I understand you hear voices, but I do not hear them." "That sound was a car backfiring outside; it wasn't gunfire." (Aids reality testing without arguing).

- **Summarizing:** Briefly restating key points of the interaction. Useful for ending sessions or transitioning topics. "So far, we've discussed your feelings about... and your plan to..." (Provides closure and confirms mutual understanding).

- **Broad Openings:** Allowing the patient to choose the topic. "What's on your mind today?" "Where would you like to begin?" (Indicates patient leads).

- **Voicing Doubt:** Gently expressing uncertainty about the reality of the patient's perceptions (especially delusions/hallucinations). "That seems hard to believe." "Really?" (Encourages patient to reconsider without direct confrontation).

Common Non-Therapeutic Blocks (Hindrances):

- **Giving Premature Advice:** Telling the patient what to do ("You should leave your job"). Negates their ability to problem-solve. Better: "What options have you considered?"

- **Minimizing Feelings:** Downplaying the patient's experience ("Everyone feels down sometimes," "It's not that bad"). Invalidating. Better: "It sounds incredibly difficult."

- **False Reassurance:** Promising outcomes you can't guarantee ("Everything will be okay," "Don't worry"). Dismisses valid concerns, can destroy trust if things don't improve. Better: "We will work through this together," "I'm here to support you."

- **Making Value Judgments:** Expressing approval or disapproval ("That's good," "You shouldn't have done that"). Implies the nurse knows best, can lead to patient trying to please the nurse rather than being authentic. Better: Remain neutral, explore consequences.

- **Asking Excessive "Why" Questions:** As mentioned, can sound accusatory. Better: Use "What" or "How."

- **Changing the Subject Inappropriately:** Shifting topics when the conversation gets uncomfortable for the nurse. Avoids dealing with important patient issues.

- **Excessive Questioning:** Bombarding the patient with questions without allowing reflection; feels like interrogation.

- **Giving Approval/Agreeing:** "That's the right decision!" Patient may feel they must always make choices the nurse approves of. Better: "What are the benefits of that decision for you?"

- **Disapproving/Disagreeing:** "That's wrong." Can make the patient defensive, block exploration. Better: "Let's look at what might happen if you do that."

- **Using Clichés or Stereotyped Comments:** "Keep your chin up," "Every cloud has a silver lining." Trite, dismissive.

Quick Reference: Do vs. Don't

DO (Therapeutic)	DON'T (Non-Therapeutic)

Offer Self	Give Premature Advice
Use Silence	Minimize Feelings
Make Observations	Give False Reassurance
Reflect Feelings/Content	Make Value Judgments (Approve/Disapprove)
Restate/Paraphrase	Ask Excessive "Why" Questions
Seek Clarification	Change Subject Inappropriately
Focus	Ask Excessive Questions (Interrogate)
Present Reality (cautiously)	Use Clichés/Stereotypes
Summarize	Agree/Disagree Excessively
Use Broad Openings	
Voice Doubt (gently)	

Ask Open-Ended Questions ("What"/"How")	

Communicating with Anxious Depressed or Psychotic Patients

While the core principles apply to everyone, communication often needs tailoring based on the patient's primary symptoms.

Communicating with an Anxious Patient:

- **Goal:** Reduce anxiety, increase sense of security.

- **Approach:**

  - Maintain a **calm, quiet demeanor**. Your anxiety can increase theirs.

  - Use **clear, simple, brief** statements. Anxiety impairs concentration.

  - Be **patient**; allow them time to respond.

  - **Reduce environmental stimuli** if possible (lower lights, less noise).

  - **Acknowledge their anxiety** or fear ("You seem anxious").

  - Help them **identify the source** of anxiety if possible ("What are you feeling right now?").

  - Focus on the **here and now**.

  - Teach and encourage **coping mechanisms** (deep breathing, relaxation).

  - Provide **reassurance about safety** if needed, but avoid false reassurance about outcomes.

Communicating with a Depressed Patient:

- **Goal:** Instill hope (without false reassurance), build self-esteem, encourage expression of feelings (even negative ones).

- **Approach:**

    o Be **patient and allow silence**. They may have psychomotor slowing and difficulty concentrating.

    o Use a **calm, accepting** approach. Avoid excessive cheerfulness, which can feel invalidating.

    o **Acknowledge their pain** or sadness ("It sounds like you're in a very dark place").

    o Spend **short, frequent periods** with withdrawn patients ("I'll sit with you for 10 minutes"). Consistency is key.

    o Focus on **small, achievable steps** or goals. Recognize and reinforce any effort.

    o If suicidal thoughts are suspected, **ask directly** ("Are you thinking about harming yourself?"). This does *not* plant the idea.

    o Help them identify **negative thought patterns** gently (linking to cognitive model).

    o Encourage participation in activities but **don't push too hard**. Start small.

Communicating with a Patient Experiencing Psychosis (e.g., Schizophrenia):

- **Goal:** Decrease anxiety, increase reality testing, ensure safety, build trust.

- **Approach:**

- Be **calm, consistent, and predictable**.

- Use **clear, concrete, simple language**. Avoid abstract ideas or metaphors.

- **Speak relatively briefly**. Impaired attention is common.

- **Maintain eye contact** without staring (monitor for paranoia).

- **Do not argue with delusions or hallucinations.** Arguing entrenches the belief and damages rapport.

- **Acknowledge the patient's *experience* or *feeling* without validating the *content*.** "It sounds frightening to hear those voices," (Validates fear) NOT "Those voices are real."

- **Gently present reality.** "I don't hear the voices, but I understand you do." "I am your nurse; I am not part of the FBI."

- **Focus on reality-based topics** and activities. Redirect away from delusional content if possible. "Let's talk about the schedule for group today."

- **Identify triggers** that increase anxiety or symptoms.

- **Ensure safety** (monitor for command hallucinations urging harm).

- **Set limits** on disruptive behavior clearly and calmly.

Practice Scenario Analysis

- *Scenario:* A patient with schizophrenia says, "The spiders are crawling on my skin! Get them off!"

  - *Non-Therapeutic Response:* "There are no spiders on you. Stop imagining things!" (Dismissive, argues with perception).

  - *Therapeutic Response:* "That sounds like a very frightening and uncomfortable feeling, like spiders are on your skin. I don't see any spiders, but I can see you are scared. Let's focus on your breathing together." (Acknowledges feeling, presents reality gently, offers coping strategy, ensures safety focus).

Moving Words Wisely

Therapeutic communication is a skill refined over a lifetime of practice. It demands constant self-awareness — recognizing not only the patient's responses but also our own internal reactions and biases. It involves choosing words carefully, listening intently, and understanding that sometimes the most therapeutic thing we can do is simply be present in silence. These techniques are your tools; learning to use them wisely and compassionately is central to effective mental health nursing. Having established the importance of relationship and communication, we now turn to a fundamental assessment tool that relies heavily on these skills: the Mental Status Examination.

Core Learnings from This Section

- **Therapeutic Communication** is purposeful interaction aimed at meeting patient needs.

- **Active Listening** (being present, observing, reflecting) is foundational.

- Use **open-ended questions** for exploration, **closed-ended** for specific facts, and **clarifying questions** for understanding. Avoid "Why?" questions.

- Employ **therapeutic techniques** (offering self, reflecting, summarizing, etc.) to facilitate communication.

- Recognize and avoid **non-therapeutic blocks** (advice-giving, false reassurance, minimizing, etc.) that hinder progress.

- **Tailor communication** based on patient symptoms (anxiety, depression, psychosis) while maintaining core principles.

- Effective communication requires practice, self-awareness, and skill.

Chapter 4: The Mental Status Examination MSE Made Easy

The Mental Status Examination, or MSE, is the cornerstone of psychiatric assessment. Think of it as the psychological equivalent of a physical exam—a systematic way to observe and describe a patient's current mental state. It's not about diagnosing; it's about gathering objective and subjective data regarding thoughts, feelings, and behaviors *at a specific point in time*. Mastering the MSE provides a snapshot of functioning that helps inform nursing diagnoses, plan care, and track changes over time. It might seem daunting initially, but breaking it down into components makes it manageable and an indispensable tool in your nursing kit.

Purpose and Components

Purpose: The primary purpose of the MSE is to obtain a baseline assessment of a patient's mental functioning across several domains. This baseline helps to:

- Identify areas of concern or dysfunction.

- Inform nursing diagnoses and care planning.

- Monitor changes in mental status over time (e.g., response to medication, worsening of symptoms).

- Communicate findings clearly and concisely to the interprofessional team.

Components: While different mnemonics exist, a common and useful one is **ASEPTIC** (or similar variations like **ABSEPTIC**). Let's use **A**ppearance, **B**ehavior, **S**peech, **E**motion (Mood/Affect), **P**erception, **T**hought Content/Process, **I**nsight/Judgment, and **C**ognition. We will explore each.

Appearance and Behavior

This section captures your objective observations of how the patient looks and acts during the assessment.

- **Appearance:**
    - **Apparent Age:** Do they look their stated age? Older? Younger?
    - **Dress:** Appropriate for age, setting, weather? Clean, neat, meticulous, disheveled, bizarre, seductive?
    - **Grooming & Hygiene:** Well-groomed, adequate, poor, malodorous? Evidence of self-neglect?
    - **Physical Characteristics:** Notable features, signs of injury, physical illness, nutritional status (well-nourished, thin, obese).

- **Behavior (Motor Activity):**
    - **Level of Activity:** Psychomotor retardation (slowed movements), agitation (restlessness, pacing), normal activity level.
    - **Type of Activity:** Purposeful, restless, bizarre, stereotyped (repetitive, non-goal-directed movements).
    - **Gait & Posture:** Stiff, shuffling, slumped, upright, unusual gait.
    - **Eye Contact:** Good, fair, poor, avoidant, intense/staring.
    - **Mannerisms/Gestures:** Tremors, tics, lip-smacking, hand-wringing, ritualistic behaviors, combativeness, rigidity.

- **Attitude Toward Examiner:** Cooperative, guarded, suspicious, hostile, friendly, seductive, indifferent, withdrawn, attentive.

Example Description: *"Patient appears stated age of 32. Dressed in clean but mismatched clothing, inappropriate for warm weather (wearing heavy coat indoors). Fair grooming with noticeable body odor. Appears thin. Behaviorally, exhibits psychomotor agitation, pacing the room rapidly and unable to sit still. Eye contact is fleeting. Frequently wrings hands. Cooperative but guarded during interaction."*

Speech

This focuses on the *mechanics* of speech, not the content (which comes later).

- **Rate:** Slow, hesitant, normal, rapid, pressured (rapid, difficult to interrupt).

- **Volume:** Soft, whispered, normal, loud, shouting.

- **Rhythm/Fluency:** Monotone, hesitant, stuttering, smooth, articulate, slurred, mumbled.

- **Quantity:** Poverty of speech (minimal responses), laconic (brief, concise), normal, verbose/talkative, spontaneous, non-spontaneous (only responds to questions).

Example Description: *"Speech is pressured and rapid in rate, loud volume. Difficult to interrupt. Quantity is verbose, flowing spontaneously."* OR *"Speech is slow, hesitant, soft volume. Quantity demonstrates poverty of speech, often responding only 'yes' or 'no'."*

Emotion Mood and Affect

This crucial section assesses the patient's emotional state. Mood and Affect are related but distinct.

- **Mood:** The patient's **subjective, sustained** emotional state, as reported by them. Ask: "How has your mood been?" "How are you feeling inside?" Document using the patient's own words in quotes if possible.

    - *Descriptors:* Euthymic (normal/stable), depressed, sad, anxious, irritable, angry, euphoric (exaggerated happiness), elated, dysphoric (unpleasant unease).

- **Affect:** The **objective, observed** expression of emotion through facial expression, tone of voice, and body language. This is what *you* see.

    - *Range/Intensity:* Full/Broad (normal variation), constricted/restricted (limited variation), blunted (minimal expression), flat (absent expression).

    - *Appropriateness:* Is the affect congruent (matching) or incongruent (not matching) the stated mood or situation? (e.g., laughing while describing a tragedy is incongruent).

    - *Lability:* Rapid shifts in affect that may seem unrelated to external stimuli.

Example Description: *"Mood reported as 'depressed and hopeless.' Affect observed as flat, with minimal facial expression and monotonous tone of voice. Affect is congruent with stated mood."* OR *"Mood described as 'on top of the world!' Affect is labile, shifting rapidly from laughter to tears during the interview, and incongruent with thought content at times."*

Perception

This assesses how the patient is experiencing the world through their senses. Disturbances here are hallmarks of psychosis but can occur in other conditions (e.g., delirium, substance withdrawal).

- **Hallucinations:** False sensory perceptions *without* real external stimuli. Ask directly but non-judgmentally: "Do you ever hear things others don't hear?" "See things others don't see?" "Feel strange sensations on your skin?"

    - *Auditory:* Hearing voices (most common), clicks, noises. Specify if command hallucinations (voices telling them to do something - assess for dangerous commands).

    - *Visual:* Seeing people, objects, lights, shapes not present.

    - *Tactile:* Feeling things on the skin (e.g., bugs crawling - formication).

    - *Olfactory:* Smelling odors not present.

    - *Gustatory:* Tasting things not present.

- **Illusions:** Misinterpretations of *real* external stimuli. (e.g., seeing faces in patterns on the floor, mistaking shadows for people). Ask: "Do things ever look different or strange to you?"

- **Derealization:** Feeling that the external world is strange or unreal.

- **Depersonalization:** Feeling detached from oneself or that one's body is unreal.

Example Description: *"Denies visual, tactile, olfactory, gustatory hallucinations. Admits to auditory hallucinations: 'hearing voices arguing' occurring intermittently throughout the day. Denies command hallucinations. Reports sometimes 'things look wavy' (possible illusion). Denies derealization/depersonalization."*

Thought Content and Process

This examines *what* the patient thinks about (content) and *how* they organize their thoughts (process).

- **Thought Content (What they think):**
  - **Suicidal or Homicidal Ideation (SI/HI):** Always assess directly. "Are you having thoughts of harming yourself?" "Thoughts of harming others?" If yes, assess plan, intent, means.
  - **Delusions:** Fixed, false beliefs held despite evidence to the contrary, not shared by culture.
    - *Persecutory:* Believing one is being watched, harmed, plotted against.
    - *Grandiose:* Inflated sense of self-worth, power, knowledge, identity.
    - *Somatic:* Belief about bodily function or defect (e.g., rotting insides).
    - *Reference:* Believing external events have special personal meaning (e.g., TV talking directly to them).
    - *Control:* Belief one's thoughts/actions are controlled by external forces (thought insertion/withdrawal/broadcasting).
    - *Nihilistic:* Belief self or world doesn't exist or is ending.
  - **Obsessions:** Persistent, intrusive thoughts, ideas, or images causing anxiety.
  - **Phobias:** Irrational fears of specific objects or situations.
  - **Religiosity:** Preoccupation with religious themes (assess if change from baseline).

75

- o **Poverty of Content:** Speech that is adequate in amount but conveys little information.

- **Thought Process (How they think):** Observe the flow and organization of speech.

  - o **Normal:** Logical, linear, coherent, goal-directed.

  - o **Circumstantiality:** Indirect, delayed reaching the point due to excessive, irrelevant detail, but *eventually gets back* to the point.

  - o **Tangentiality:** Wanders off topic and *never returns* to the original point.

  - o **Loose Associations (Derailment):** Illogical shifting between unrelated topics. Ideas slip off track.

  - o **Flight of Ideas:** Rapid shifting of topics with only superficial connections, often seen in mania; speech may be pressured.

  - o **Word Salad:** Incoherent mixture of random words and phrases.

  - o **Neologisms:** Made-up words meaningful only to the patient.

  - o **Clang Associations:** Speaking in rhymes or based on sound rather than meaning.

  - o **Thought Blocking:** Sudden interruption in speech or train of thought before completion.

  - o **Perseveration:** Repeating the same word, phrase, or idea.

Example Description: *"Thought content reveals persecutory delusions ('neighbors spying with cameras') and denies SI/HI. Thought process is tangential, frequently losing the thread of* conversation. Some loose associations noted. Denies obsessions/phobias." OR "Thought content significant for grandiose delusions ('invented the internet'). Admits to fleeting suicidal thoughts without plan or intent. Thought process demonstrates flight of ideas, difficult to follow conversation due to rapid topic shifts. Clang associations present ('sky high buy fly')."

Insight and Judgment

These assess the patient's awareness and decision-making abilities.

- **Insight:** Awareness and understanding of one's own illness, symptoms, and situation.
    - *Full:* Recognizes illness, symptoms, and need for treatment.
    - *Partial:* Admits illness but attributes symptoms to external factors, or uncertain about need for treatment.
    - *Poor/Absent:* Denies illness or symptoms altogether.
- **Judgment:** Ability to make sound decisions, understand consequences of actions, and act appropriately in social situations. Assess by observing choices during hospitalization, or posing hypothetical scenarios ("What would you do if you found a stamped, addressed envelope on the street?").
    - *Good:* Makes decisions that consider consequences and safety.
    - *Fair:* Able to make reasonable decisions but may need prompting.

- *Poor:* Makes decisions that are impulsive, unsafe, or disregard consequences.

Example Description: *"Insight is poor; patient denies having depression, states 'I'm just tired.' Judgment appears fair; able to state appropriate action in hypothetical scenario but struggles with applying planning to current situation."* OR *"Insight is full; patient recognizes bipolar disorder, links current mania to stopping medication. Judgment is impaired related to mania, evidenced by recent excessive spending and impulsive travel plans."*[46]

Cognition

This assesses basic brain functions like orientation, memory, and attention. Formal neuropsychological testing is more detailed, but the MSE provides a screen.

- **Orientation:** Awareness of Person, Place, Time, and Situation (Ox4). Ask: "What is your name?" "Where are you right now (hospital name/city)?" "What is today's date (day, month, year)?" "Why are you here?"

- **Memory:**

  - *Immediate:* Recall 3 unrelated words immediately after hearing them.

  - *Recent:* Recall the same 3 words after 5 minutes. Recall events of the past few days/week.

  - *Remote:* Recall distant events (verifiable if possible, e.g., birthday, past presidents, significant historical events).

- **Concentration/Attention:** Ability to focus and sustain attention.

  - *Serial 7s:* Subtract 7 from 100, then 7 from that result, etc. (Note effort and accuracy).

- o *Spell WORLD backward.*
- o Observe ability to attend during the interview.

Example Description: *"Cognition: Oriented x 4. Immediate recall 3/3 words, recent recall 2/3 words after 5 minutes. Remote memory intact for date of birth. Concentration fair; able to subtract serial 7s twice correctly with effort before losing track. Able to spell WORLD backward."*

How to Conduct and Document the MSE Concisely

- **Integrate into Conversation:** Don't administer the MSE like a rigid checklist. Weave questions and observations into your natural therapeutic conversation and assessment. Much information (appearance, behavior, speech, affect) is gathered through simple observation while talking.

- **Be Flexible:** Adjust the depth based on the patient's condition and cooperativeness. A full cognitive screen might not be feasible with someone acutely psychotic or severely depressed.

- **Use Objective Language:** Describe what you see and hear. Avoid jargon where possible, but use standard MSE terms accurately. Avoid judgmental language.

- **Be Concise:** Document findings efficiently using standard terms. Focus on significant positive and negative findings. "WNL" (within normal limits) can be used judiciously for sections without abnormalities *after* a thorough assessment.

- **Document Baseline and Changes:** Note the initial MSE findings clearly. Subsequent notes should highlight any *changes* from the baseline.

MSE Checklist/Template (Conceptual - Use for Note-Taking/Guidance)

(Not for direct patient use, but helps organize thoughts/documentation)

- **Appearance:** Apparent age, Dress, Grooming/Hygiene, Physical features.

- **Behavior:** Motor activity level/type, Gait/Posture, Eye contact, Mannerisms, Attitude.

- **Speech:** Rate, Volume, Rhythm, Quantity.

- **Emotion:**

  - Mood: (Patient's report - use quotes).

  - Affect: Range (full, constricted, flat), Appropriateness (congruent/incongruent), Lability.

- **Perception:** Hallucinations (Auditory, Visual, Tactile, Olfactory, Gustatory - specify type/content if present), Illusions, Derealization/Depersonalization. (Note denials).

- **Thought Content:** SI/HI (assess plan/intent if present), Delusions (type/theme), Obsessions, Phobias, Other preoccupations. (Note denials).

- **Thought Process:** Coherent, Logical, Circumstantial, Tangential, Loose Associations, Flight of Ideas, Blocking, Perseveration, etc.

- **Insight:** Full, Partial, Poor.

- **Judgment:** Good, Fair, Poor (provide evidence if poor).

- **Cognition:**

- Orientation: (Person, Place, Time, Situation - Ox?).

- Memory: Immediate (/3), Recent (/3), Remote.

- Concentration: (Serial 7s, WORLD backward, Observed attention).

Example of Concise Documentation:

"Pt is 48yo male, appears stated age, casually dressed, fair hygiene. Psychomotor activity WNL. Cooperative, maintains fair eye contact. Speech normal rate/volume. Mood 'okay'. Affect constricted, congruent. Denies hallucinations/illusions. Denies SI/HI. Thought process linear/coherent. No delusions apparent. Insight partial ('Maybe stress is getting to me'). Judgment fair. Oriented x4. Immediate/recent recall 3/3. Concentration intact. MSE reveals constricted affect and partial insight as main findings currently."

Observations as Foundation

The Mental Status Examination is your primary tool for systematically observing and documenting a patient's mental state at a given moment. It requires keen observation skills, effective communication to elicit information, and precise language to record your findings. While parts of it might feel like a checklist, remember it flows best when integrated into a therapeutic conversation. The data gathered forms the bedrock upon which nursing diagnoses are made and care is planned. It's a dynamic assessment—always be ready to compare today's findings with yesterday's baseline to track progress or identify emerging concerns. With practice, the MSE becomes an intuitive and essential part of your nursing assessment repertoire.

Core Learnings from This Section

- The **MSE** is a systematic assessment of current mental functioning, like a psychological physical exam.

- Key components include **A**ppearance, **B**ehavior, **S**peech, **E**motion (Mood/Affect), **P**erception, **T**hought Content/Process, **I**nsight/Judgment, **C**ognition (**ABSEPTIC** mnemonic).

- Assess each component through **observation** and **direct questioning**, integrating it into the conversation.

- Use **objective, descriptive language** and standard terminology for documentation.

- Distinguish **Mood** (subjective report) from **Affect** (objective observation).

- Assess **Thought Content** (what) and **Thought Process** (how).

- Always assess for **suicidal/homicidal ideation** directly.

- **Insight** (awareness) and **Judgment** (decision-making) are critical components.

- The MSE provides a **baseline** and helps track changes over time.

Chapter 5:Safety and Risk Assessment Essentials

Our primary commitment, woven into the very fabric of nursing ethics, is to protect those in our care from harm—and sometimes, to protect others from potential harm as well. In mental health settings, where individuals may be struggling with intense emotional pain, distorted thinking, overwhelming impulses, or profound despair, this commitment takes on particular urgency. Assessing risk isn't about predicting the future with a crystal ball; it's about systematically gathering information, recognizing warning signs, understanding vulnerabilities, and implementing thoughtful interventions to mitigate danger and support well-being. It requires sharp observation, sensitive communication, and sound clinical judgment.

Identifying Risk Factors Understanding Vulnerabilities

Recognizing factors associated with increased risk helps us know when to heighten our vigilance and focus our assessment. These factors don't *guarantee* an adverse event will happen, but they signal increased vulnerability. We often think about risk in three main categories: harm to self (suicide), non-suicidal self-injury, and harm to others.

Risk Factors for Suicide: Suicide is complex, arising from an interaction of many factors. Knowing these helps guide our assessment:

- **Mental Disorders:** The strongest link. Especially Mood Disorders (MDD, Bipolar), Schizophrenia, Substance Use Disorders, Anxiety Disorders, PTSD, Borderline Personality Disorder, Antisocial Personality Disorder. Co-occurring disorders increase risk.

- **Previous Suicide Attempt(s):** This is one of the strongest predictors of future attempts. Always ask about past attempts, their lethality, and circumstances.

- **Hopelessness:** A pervasive sense that things will never get better. This feeling is often more predictive than the depth of depression itself. Listen for statements of despair, futility.

- **Suicidal Ideation, Plan, Intent:** Current thoughts of death, specific plans (how, when, where), and the stated intent to act on those plans signal escalating risk.

- **Access to Lethal Means:** Availability of firearms, medications, ligatures, etc., significantly increases the risk that ideation will become action.

- **History of Trauma or Abuse:** Childhood abuse, combat exposure, sexual assault increase vulnerability.

- **Substance Use/Abuse:** Lowers inhibitions, impairs judgment, can worsen depression/psychosis, and is involved in many suicides. Acute intoxication or withdrawal are high-risk periods.

- **Recent Losses or Stressors:** Relationship breakup, death of loved one, job loss, financial crisis, legal trouble, serious illness diagnosis.

- **Social Isolation/Lack of Support:** Feeling alone, disconnected from family, friends, community.

- **Chronic Physical Illness/Pain:** Especially conditions that are debilitating or life-limiting.

- **Impulsivity/Agitation/Severe Anxiety:** Can increase the likelihood of acting on suicidal thoughts without deliberation. Sometimes, a sudden increase in energy in a depressed person can precede an attempt.

- **Family History:** Family history of suicide, mental illness, or substance abuse.

- **Demographics (Use with Caution):** Statistically, certain groups have higher rates (e.g., older males, specific Indigenous populations, LGBTQ+ youth facing rejection), but individual risk assessment is always paramount – demographics alone tell you little about a specific person.

Risk Factors for Non-Suicidal Self-Injury (NSSI): NSSI (e.g., cutting, burning, hitting oneself) is typically done to cope with intense emotional pain, feelings of emptiness, or dissociation, **without** the intent to die (though risk of accidental death exists, and it's a risk factor for future suicide attempts).

- **Mental Disorders:** Strongly associated with BPD, also seen in depression, anxiety, PTSD, eating disorders.

- **History of Trauma/Abuse:** Very common.

- **Emotional Dysregulation:** Difficulty managing intense emotions.

- **Low Self-Esteem/Self-Criticism.**

- **Social Isolation or Difficult Peer Relationships.**

- **History of NSSI:** Past behavior predicts future behavior.

- **Impulsivity.**

Risk Factors for Harm to Others (Aggression/Violence): While the vast majority of people with mental illness are *not* violent and are more likely to be victims, a small subset may pose a risk. Predicting violence is difficult, but certain factors increase concern:

- **Past History of Violence:** This is the single best predictor of future violence. Always assess history thoroughly.

- **Substance Use/Intoxication:** Strongly associated with increased aggression (especially alcohol, stimulants, PCP). Withdrawal can also increase irritability.

- **Certain Psychiatric Symptoms:**
    - *Command Hallucinations:* Voices telling the person to harm someone (assess content, intent to obey).
    - *Paranoid Delusions:* Belief others intend harm can lead to preemptive aggression.
    - *Mania:* Impulsivity, irritability, poor judgment can lower threshold for aggression.
    - *Antisocial Personality Disorder:* Disregard for others, history of aggression.
    - *Intermittent Explosive Disorder.*

- **Impulsivity/Poor Emotional Control.**

- **Neurological Impairment:** Traumatic brain injury, certain dementias.

- **Feeling Threatened or Provoked:** Perception matters; someone feeling cornered or disrespected may react aggressively.

- **Access to Weapons.**

- **Younger Male Demographics:** Statistically higher rates, but again, individual assessment is key.

Risk Factor Summary (Text List):

- **Suicide:** Mental illness (esp. mood disorders, psychosis, SUDs), prior attempts, hopelessness, ideation/plan/intent, access to means, trauma hx, substance use, recent loss, isolation, chronic illness, impulsivity/agitation, family hx.

- **NSSI:** Mental illness (esp. BPD), trauma hx, emotional dysregulation, low self-esteem, isolation, past NSSI, impulsivity.

- **Harm to Others:** Past violence, substance use, command hallucinations/paranoia, mania, ASPD, impulsivity, feeling threatened, access to weapons.

Key Assessment Questions The Courage to Ask

Assessing risk isn't passive; it requires direct, specific questioning within a supportive, non-judgmental therapeutic relationship. Avoiding these questions out of discomfort does a grave disservice to the patient. Building rapport first helps, but don't let rapport-building delay essential safety questions if risk seems high.

Assessing Suicidal Ideation (SI):

- Start broad, then get specific. "How have your spirits been lately?" "Have things felt hopeless or like life isn't worth living?"

- **Ask Directly:** "Are you having thoughts of hurting yourself?" "Are you thinking about ending your life?" "Have you wished you were dead?" (Use language the patient can understand).

- **If Yes to Ideation:**

    o **Frequency/Intensity/Duration:** "How often do these thoughts occur?" "How strong are they?" "How long do they last?"

    o **Plan:** "Have you thought about how you might do this?" (Ask for details – method, time, place). The more specific the plan, the higher the risk.

- o **Means:** "Do you have access to [the method mentioned - pills, weapon, etc.]?" "Where is [the means] now?"

- o **Intent:** "How likely do you think you are to act on these thoughts?" "What stops you?" (Identify protective factors). "On a scale of 0-10, how strong is your intention to kill yourself right now?"

- o **Past Attempts:** "Have you ever tried to harm yourself or end your life before?" (Ask about methods, circumstances, medical severity).

- o **Rehearsal:** "Have you practiced or taken any steps toward carrying out your plan?" (e.g., writing a note, acquiring means).

Assessing Non-Suicidal Self-Injury (NSSI):

- Ask directly but sensitively. "Sometimes when people feel overwhelmed, they do things to hurt themselves on the outside to cope with pain on the inside. Is this something you've experienced?"

- **If Yes:**

  - o **Methods:** "What methods do you use?"

  - o **Frequency/Triggers:** "How often does this happen?" "What usually leads up to it?" "What are you feeling right before/during/after?"

  - o **Purpose/Function:** "What does doing this do for you?" (e.g., "Does it help you feel relief?" "Feel something other than numb?" "Punish yourself?"). Understanding the function guides interventions.

- Severity/Medical Risk: Assess severity of injury, need for medical attention.

- Distinguish from Suicidal Intent: "When you hurt yourself, are you intending to end your life, or is it more about coping with feelings?" (Though acknowledge overlap/risk).

Assessing Harm to Others:

- Assess anger, irritability, frustration levels. "How have you been managing your anger lately?"

- Ask about history of violence directly. "Have you ever gotten into physical fights?" "Have you ever hurt someone else or damaged property when angry?"

- Ask about current thoughts/urges. "Are you having thoughts of harming anyone right now?"

- **If Yes:**

  - Target: "Who are you thinking of harming?" (Identify potential victim).

  - Plan: "Have you thought about how you might do it?"

  - Intent: "How likely are you to act on these thoughts?"

  - Means: "Do you have access to weapons?"

  - Command Hallucinations: "Are voices telling you to harm someone?" "What are they saying?" "Do you feel you have to obey them?"

General Approach to Risk Assessment Questioning:

- **Normalize:** Frame questions non-judgmentally ("Sometimes when people feel as down as you do, they have thoughts of death...").

- **Be Direct:** Don't beat around the bush with safety questions.

- **Listen Actively:** Pay attention to verbal content, nonverbal cues, and emotional tone.

- **Validate Feelings:** Acknowledge the pain or distress underlying the thoughts ("It sounds like you're in incredible pain right now").

- **Document Thoroughly:** Record questions asked, patient's specific responses (use quotes), your assessment of risk level, and rationale.

"Safety First" Tip Box: Asking directly about suicide does **NOT** plant the idea in someone's head. It opens the door for them to talk about it and allows you to intervene. Silence is far more dangerous.

Safety Planning Basics A Collaborative Lifeline

When a patient expresses suicidal ideation or significant urges for self-harm, developing a **Safety Plan** *with them* is a key intervention. It's not a "no-suicide contract" (which have limited effectiveness and can create false reassurance). Instead, it's a collaboratively written document outlining concrete steps the person can take to stay safe during a crisis. It empowers the patient by focusing on their strengths and resources.

Key Components of a Safety Plan:

1. **Recognizing Warning Signs:** Helping the patient identify their personal triggers and early warning signs (specific thoughts, moods, physical feelings, behaviors, or situations) that indicate a crisis might be developing or

escalating. *Examples: Feeling overwhelming hopelessness, isolating oneself, increased substance use urge, specific anniversaries.*

2. **Internal Coping Strategies:** Things the patient can do *on their own* to distract themselves or cope without contacting anyone else. *Examples: Listening to specific music, deep breathing, mindfulness exercises, taking a walk, watching a specific movie, engaging in a hobby, journaling.* These should be realistic and accessible.

3. **People and Social Settings for Distraction:** Identifying specific people or safe public places that can help distract from distressing thoughts or urges. *Examples: Calling a specific friend (to talk about unrelated things), going to a coffee shop, visiting a library or park.*

4. **People to Ask for Help:** Listing specific family members, friends, or other trusted supports the patient can reach out to for help when coping strategies aren't enough. Include phone numbers. Discuss *how* to ask for help.

5. **Professional Help Contacts:** Listing names and numbers of therapists, psychiatrists, clinics, local crisis lines (e.g., National Suicide Prevention Lifeline - 988 in US), or emergency services (911/999). Explicitly stating when to use each level of support.

6. **Making the Environment Safe:** Identifying and limiting access to lethal means identified during the risk assessment (e.g., giving firearms to a trusted person, discarding excess medications). This is a critical, evidence-based part of reducing risk.

Nurse's Role in Safety Planning:

- **Collaborate:** Develop the plan *with* the patient, using their words and ideas. It must feel owned by them.

- **Be Specific & Concrete:** Avoid vague suggestions. List specific names, numbers, activities.

- **Assess Feasibility:** Ensure the planned coping strategies and supports are realistic and accessible for the patient.

- **Provide a Copy:** Give the patient a written copy to keep readily available (wallet card, phone note).

- **Share (with consent):** Share the plan with family/supports and the treatment team.

- **Review & Revise:** Safety plans are living documents; review and update them regularly, especially if risk level changes or coping strategies prove ineffective.

Safety planning doesn't eliminate risk, but it provides a concrete roadmap for managing crises, instills hope by focusing on resources, and strengthens the therapeutic alliance.

Case Snippet: Safety Planning

- *Scenario:* Maria, assessed as having moderate suicide risk with recent ideation but no specific plan, agrees to work on a safety plan with her nurse, Sam.

- *Nursing Action:* Sam sits with Maria and guides her through the steps. Maria identifies feeling intensely lonely and starting to think "it's too much" as warning signs (Step 1). For internal coping, she identifies listening to calming music and doing puzzles (Step 2). She names her sister (who lives nearby) and a specific coffee shop as distractions (Step 3). She lists her sister again and a close friend as people she could call for help, writing down their numbers (Step 4). Sam ensures she has the numbers for her outpatient therapist and the local crisis line (Step 5). They discuss removing the expired prescription pain medication she mentioned having at home (Step 6). Sam writes this down clearly, gives Maria a copy, documents it, and discusses it with the team and Maria's sister (with Maria's consent).

Understanding Different Levels of Observation Keeping Watch

In inpatient settings, **observation levels** (often called "checks" or "precautions") are specific nursing interventions ordered based on assessed risk. The goal is always to use the **least restrictive** level necessary to maintain safety.

Common Levels (Specific names/intervals may vary by facility):

- **General Observation (or Routine Checks):** Staff maintain general awareness of all patients' locations and activities. Patients checked at routine intervals (e.g., every 30-60 minutes) as part of standard unit rounds. Appropriate for patients assessed as low risk.

- **Close Observation (or Q15-Minute Checks):** Requires staff to have direct line-of-sight observation of the patient at least every 15 minutes (or other specified interval). Staff must document the patient's location, behavior, and mood at each check. Used for patients at moderate risk for suicide, self-harm, aggression, elopement, or severe withdrawal. *Important:* This is not just glancing in a room; it requires visualizing the patient and assessing their immediate safety/behavior.

- **Constant Observation (1:1):** Requires a specific staff member be assigned solely to that patient, remaining within arm's length or immediate line of sight **at all times**, including during bathroom use and sleep. Used for patients at high, imminent risk of harm to self (e.g., active suicidal plan/intent) or others (e.g., acute aggression). This is highly restrictive and requires clear documentation of rationale and frequent reassessment. The observing staff member must be vigilant and focused solely on the assigned patient. Therapeutic engagement during 1:1 is encouraged when appropriate, but safety monitoring is the priority.

- **Line of Sight Observation:** Similar to 1:1, but staff must keep the patient in view at all times, though perhaps not always within arm's length (e.g., patient can be across the room but must be visible).

Nursing Considerations for Observations:

- Observation level is based on ongoing **risk assessment**, not diagnosis.

- Clearly **communicate** the assigned level to all staff (report, assignment sheets).

- Perform checks **purposefully** and **reliably**. Don't sign off without actually observing.

- **Document** each check according to policy (time, location, behavior, mood, signature).

- **Engage therapeutically** during checks when possible ("How are you feeling right now, Mr. Smith?"). Checks are safety measures, but also opportunities for interaction.

- **Reassess frequently** (at least every shift and PRN) if the current level is still necessary. Advocate for reducing the level as risk decreases to maintain the least restrictive environment.

- Provide **clear explanations** to the patient (and family, if appropriate) about why observations are needed, framing it as a safety measure.

The Therapeutic Milieu and Environmental Safety The Safe Container

The **therapeutic milieu** refers to the overall environment of the treatment setting—the physical space, the daily structure and routine, the social interactions between patients and staff, and the overall emotional atmosphere. Creating and maintaining a **safe milieu** is a constant nursing responsibility.

Key Aspects of Environmental Safety:

- **Physical Environment Design:** Modern units aim for safety features:
    - Anti-ligature fixtures (door handles, shower heads, faucets designed to prevent hanging).
    - Shatterproof glass/windows.
    - Locked windows, secured screens.
    - Doors opening outward (prevent barricading).
    - Continuous hinges on doors.
    - Furniture that is heavy or difficult to throw/break.
    - Good visibility (clear sightlines in common areas, observation windows).
    - Secure nursing station.
- **Hazard Identification & Removal:** Staff must be vigilant in identifying and removing potential hazards:
    - **Routine Environmental Checks:** Regularly inspecting patient rooms, bathrooms, common areas for dangerous items.
    - **Patient Belongings Search:** Searching personal items upon admission and return from pass, per policy, to remove contraband (weapons, drugs, alcohol, medications) and potentially harmful

items (sharps, belts, cords, plastic bags, glass items, sometimes even specific clothing items). Explain the rationale clearly to patients.

- o **Monitoring Items Brought by Visitors:** Ensuring visitors don't inadvertently or intentionally bring unsafe items onto the unit.

- o **Securing Unit:** Keeping doors locked as required, monitoring entry/exit.

- **Staff Awareness and Presence:**

  - o Knowing who is on the unit and where they are.

  - o Maintaining visibility in common areas.

  - o Observing patient interactions for signs of tension or escalation.

  - o Conducting regular unit rounds.

- **Managing Milieu Dynamics:**

  - o Setting clear expectations and rules for behavior.

  - o Facilitating positive peer interactions.

  - o Intervening early to de-escalate conflicts between patients.

  - o Providing structure through scheduled groups and activities.

Nurse's Role: Active participation in environmental checks, enforcing safety policies consistently, maintaining situational awareness, intervening proactively to manage milieu dynamics, reporting safety concerns promptly, and contributing to an overall atmosphere of safety and respect.

"Safety First" Tip Box: Environmental safety isn't just about removing objects. It's also about creating a *psychologically* safe space through consistent routines, clear communication, respectful interactions, and predictable staff responses.

Vigilance Tempered with Hope

Ensuring safety is perhaps the most demanding, yet most fundamental, aspect of mental health nursing. It requires constant vigilance, astute assessment skills, the courage to ask difficult questions, the ability to act decisively in emergencies, and the wisdom to balance necessary precautions with the patient's need for autonomy and dignity. From identifying risk factors and conducting thorough assessments, to collaborative safety planning, implementing appropriate observation levels, and maintaining a secure therapeutic environment—every action is geared towards creating a space where individuals feel protected enough to begin the work of healing. It's a heavy responsibility, but one undertaken with the knowledge that safety is the bedrock upon which recovery is built.

Core Learnings from This Section

- **Safety** is the paramount priority in mental health nursing, forming the foundation for trust and therapy.

- **Risk Assessment** involves identifying **risk factors** (for suicide, NSSI, harm to others) and conducting **direct, specific questioning** regarding ideation, plans, intent, and history. Ask directly!

- **Safety Planning** is a **collaborative** intervention outlining warning signs, coping strategies, supports, and means restriction to help manage crises.

- **Observation Levels** (e.g., q15min checks, 1:1) are safety interventions based on assessed risk; use the least restrictive level needed and reassess frequently.

- Maintaining a safe **Therapeutic Milieu** involves managing the physical environment (hazard checks, unit design) and psychosocial dynamics (structure, rules, staff presence).

- Ongoing vigilance, thorough documentation, and a team approach are essential for safety.

Part 2: Understanding Common Mental Health Conditions

Chapter 6: Anxiety OCD and Related Disorders

Everyone feels anxious sometimes—it's a normal human response to stress or danger. But when anxiety becomes excessive, persistent, and interferes with daily life, it crosses the line into an anxiety *disorder*. These are among the most common mental health conditions, and they manifest in various ways, from constant worry to sudden terror to repetitive, intrusive thoughts and actions. Understanding these different presentations is key to providing effective nursing care.

Generalized Anxiety Disorder GAD

Imagine worrying intensely about *everything*—your job performance, your health, your family's safety, finances, even minor matters like being late for an appointment—most days, for months on end. This worry is pervasive, difficult to control, and out of proportion to the actual likelihood or impact of the feared events. This is the core of **Generalized Anxiety Disorder (GAD)**. It's not just stress; it's a chronic state of high anxiety and apprehension accompanied by physical symptoms.

Key Symptoms: Beyond the excessive worry, look for at least three of these physical or cognitive symptoms (for adults, present more days than not for at least 6 months):

- **Restlessness** or feeling keyed up/on edge.

- Being easily **fatigued**.

- **Difficulty concentrating** or mind going blank.

- **Irritability**.

- **Muscle tension**[3] (often headaches, neck/shoulder pain).

- **Sleep disturbance** (difficulty falling/staying asleep, restless sleep).

People with GAD often experience significant distress or impairment in social, occupational, or other important areas of functioning. They might spend hours worrying, seek constant reassurance, avoid situations they fear will trigger worry, or struggle with procrastination due to anxiety.

Nursing Priorities:

1. **Create a Calm Environment:** Reduce stimuli. Approach the patient calmly.

2. **Therapeutic Communication:** Use active listening. Encourage verbalization of feelings and worries without judgment. Avoid minimizing their concerns ("Don't worry so much"). Ask open-ended questions to understand their specific fears.

3. **Teach Coping Skills:** Relaxation techniques (deep breathing, progressive muscle relaxation), mindfulness, stress management strategies. Help them identify triggers for anxiety.

4. **Cognitive Approaches:** Help patients identify and challenge their anxious thoughts (e.g., "What's the evidence for that worry?" "What's the worst that could happen, and could I cope?"). This aligns with Cognitive Behavioral Therapy (CBT) principles.

5. **Medication Education:** Explain the purpose, dosage, side effects, and time course of any prescribed anti-anxiety medications (like SSRIs, SNRIs, or sometimes benzodiazepines for short-term use). Emphasize that medications are often most effective combined with therapy/coping skills.

6. **Promote Self-Care:** Encourage regular exercise, balanced nutrition, and good sleep hygiene, as these can impact anxiety levels.

Case Snippet: GAD

- *Scenario:* Mr. Chen, 42, presents to his primary care clinic complaining of constant headaches, neck pain, and trouble sleeping for the past year. He describes persistent worry about his job security (despite good performance reviews), his children's health (despite them being healthy), and global events he sees on the news. He feels perpetually "on edge," irritable with his family, and exhausted. He struggles to concentrate at work because his mind races with "what if" scenarios.

- *Nursing Considerations:* The clinic nurse would assess his physical symptoms but also screen for anxiety using questions about worry, concentration, sleep, and muscle tension. Priorities include validating his distress, providing education about GAD, teaching basic relaxation breathing, discussing lifestyle factors (caffeine intake, sleep habits), and reinforcing the provider's treatment plan (likely involving therapy +/- medication).

What to Watch For (GAD):

- Excessive reassurance seeking.

- Somatic complaints (headaches, GI upset, muscle aches).

- Difficulty making decisions due to worry.

- Increased substance use (attempting to self-medicate).

- Avoidance of situations perceived as stressful.

Common Nursing Diagnoses (GAD):

- **Anxiety** (moderate to severe)[7]

- **Ineffective Coping**

- **Disturbed Sleep Pattern**

- **Fatigue**
- **Readiness for Enhanced Coping** (if patient is seeking help)

Panic Disorder

Unlike the persistent hum of GAD, **Panic Disorder** involves recurrent, *unexpected* **panic attacks**. A panic attack is a sudden surge of intense fear or discomfort that peaks within minutes. It feels like terror striking out of the blue, often accompanied by overwhelming physical symptoms. The key to Panic Disorder isn't just having panic attacks (many people have one or two in their lifetime), but the persistent **fear** of having *more* attacks or worrying about their consequences (like losing control, having a heart attack, or "going crazy"). This fear often leads to significant behavioral changes, like avoiding places where attacks have occurred.

Panic Attack Symptoms (Need 4 or more during an attack):

- Palpitations, pounding heart, or accelerated heart rate.
- Sweating.
- Trembling or shaking.
- Sensations of shortness of breath or smothering.
- Feelings of choking.
- Chest pain or discomfort.
- Nausea or abdominal distress.
- Feeling dizzy, unsteady, light-headed, or faint.
- Chills or heat sensations.
- Paresthesias (numbness or tingling sensations).

- Derealization (feelings of unreality) or depersonalization (being detached from oneself).

- Fear of losing control or "going crazy."

- Fear of dying.

These attacks are terrifying precisely because they often feel like a medical emergency (heart attack, stroke, suffocation). Many people with Panic Disorder initially seek help in emergency rooms.

Nursing Priorities (During a Panic Attack):

1. **Stay with the Patient:** Do not leave them alone. Your presence provides safety and support.

2. **Maintain Calm Presence:** Speak calmly, slowly, using short, simple sentences. Be reassuring but avoid false reassurance ("You'll be fine" can feel dismissive). Try "I'm here with you. You are safe right now."

3. **Reduce Stimuli:** Move the patient to a quieter environment if possible.

4. **Coach Breathing:** Encourage slow, deep breaths. "Breathe in slowly through your nose... now out slowly through your mouth." Breathe *with* them if helpful. (Avoid encouraging deep breathing if hyperventilation is severe – sometimes breathing into cupped hands or a small paper bag briefly is needed, per protocol).

5. **Provide Brief Direction:** Give simple, concrete instructions. "Sit down here." "Focus on your breathing."

6. **Administer PRN Medication (if ordered):** Usually a fast-acting benzodiazepine. Assess effectiveness.

7. **Safety:** Ensure the patient doesn't harm themselves inadvertently during the attack (e.g., falling if dizzy).

Nursing Priorities (Between Attacks):

1. **Education:** Teach the patient about panic attacks – that they are frightening but not physically dangerous, and they *do* end. Explain the "fight or flight" response.

2. **Identify Triggers:** Help the patient recognize situations or bodily sensations that might trigger attacks (though many are unexpected).

3. **Teach Coping Skills:** Relaxation, breathing exercises, cognitive techniques (challenging catastrophic thoughts like "I'm dying").

4. **Medication Education:** Explain prescribed preventative medications (often SSRIs/SNRIs) and PRN options.

5. **Encourage Therapy:** CBT is highly effective for Panic Disorder.

Case Snippet: Panic Attack

- *Scenario:* While waiting in a crowded outpatient clinic lobby, Ms. Garcia, 28, suddenly gasps, clutches her chest, and begins trembling violently. She cries out, "I can't breathe! I think I'm having a heart attack!" Her breathing is rapid and shallow.

- *Nursing Considerations:* The triage nurse immediately recognizes a likely panic attack. Priorities: Quickly escort Ms. Garcia to a quiet exam room (staying with her), speak calmly ("Ms. Garcia, I'm right here. Let's sit down. Try to take a slow breath with me."), assess vital signs quickly to rule out acute medical issues (while recognizing panic itself elevates HR/BP), reassure her she is in a safe place, coach slow breathing. Once the attack subsides, provide education about panic symptoms and recommend follow-up assessment for Panic Disorder.

What to Watch For (Panic Disorder):

- **Agoraphobia:** Fear and avoidance of places or situations where escape might be difficult or help unavailable if a panic attack occurs (e.g., crowds, public transport, being outside alone). Can become severely disabling.

- Frequent emergency room visits.

- Anticipatory anxiety (constant worry about the *next* attack).

- Significant impact on daily routines and activities due to avoidance.

Common Nursing Diagnoses (Panic Disorder):

- **Anxiety** (severe/panic)

- **Fear** (of losing control, dying, having another attack)

- **Ineffective Breathing Pattern** (during attack)

- **Ineffective Coping**

- **Social Isolation** (if Agoraphobia develops)

Phobias

A **phobia** is an intense, persistent, irrational fear of a specific object, situation, or activity. The fear is excessive and unreasonable, recognized as such by the individual (usually), but they feel powerless to control it. Exposure to the feared stimulus provokes immediate anxiety, potentially even a panic attack.

Common Types:

- **Specific Phobia:** Fear of a particular object or situation (e.g., spiders - arachnophobia, heights - acrophobia, flying - aviophobia, injections - trypanophobia, enclosed spaces - claustrophobia).

- **Social Anxiety Disorder (Social Phobia):** Fear of social or performance situations where scrutiny by others might occur. Fear of embarrassment, humiliation, or rejection (e.g., public speaking, meeting new people, eating in public, using public restrooms). Can be generalized to most social situations or specific to performance situations.

Individuals with phobias often go to great lengths to **avoid** the feared object or situation, which significantly restricts their lives.

Nursing Priorities:

1. **Acknowledge the Fear:** Accept the patient's fear as real *to them*, even if it seems irrational to you. Avoid ridicule or forced exposure.

2. **Build Trust:** Create a safe, supportive environment.

3. **Teach Relaxation Techniques:** Deep breathing, progressive muscle relaxation can help manage anxiety when anticipating or encountering the phobic stimulus.

4. **Support Exposure Therapy (if part of treatment plan):** This is often done by therapists, but nurses can support it. It involves gradual, controlled exposure to the feared stimulus while using coping skills. The nurse might accompany a patient during an exposure exercise, provide encouragement, and reinforce coping strategies.

5. **Medication Education:** Medications (SSRIs, SNRIs, sometimes beta-blockers for performance anxiety, or benzodiazepines short-term) may be used, especially for Social Anxiety Disorder.

6. **Focus on Coping, Not Elimination:** Help the patient learn to *manage* anxiety related to the phobia, allowing them to function despite the fear.

Case Snippet: Social Phobia

- *Scenario:* John, a 19-year-old college student, reports intense anxiety about attending classes, especially seminars requiring participation. He fears saying something "stupid" and being judged. Before class, he experiences sweating, palpitations, and nausea. He has started skipping classes he perceives as high-risk for interaction.

- *Nursing Considerations:* A campus health nurse would assess the nature and severity of his anxiety, recognizing Social Anxiety Disorder. Priorities include psychoeducation about the disorder, teaching relaxation techniques to use before/during class, exploring negative self-talk related to judgment (cognitive approach), encouraging gradual steps (e.g., just attending first, then aiming to ask one question), connecting him with counseling services offering CBT/exposure therapy, and discussing potential medication options with a provider if symptoms are severe.

What to Watch For (Phobias):

- Level of avoidance behavior and its impact on daily life (job, school, relationships).

- Development of panic attacks upon exposure.

- Use of substances to cope with phobic situations.

- Social isolation (especially with Social Anxiety Disorder).

Common Nursing Diagnoses (Phobias):

- **Fear**

- **Anxiety**

- Social Isolation

- Ineffective Coping

- Impaired Social Interaction

Obsessive Compulsive Disorder OCD

Obsessive-Compulsive Disorder (OCD) is characterized by two core components:

1. **Obsessions:** Recurrent, persistent, intrusive, and unwanted thoughts, urges, or images that cause significant anxiety or distress. The person tries to ignore or suppress them, often unsuccessfully. Common themes include:

    o Contamination (germs, dirt, chemicals).

    o Need for symmetry, order, exactness.

    o Doubts (e.g., Did I lock the door? Did I hit someone with my car?).

    o Aggressive or horrific thoughts/images.

    o Sexual thoughts/images.

    o Religious concerns (scrupulosity).

2. **Compulsions:** Repetitive behaviors (e.g., hand washing, ordering, checking) or mental acts (e.g., praying, counting, repeating words[21] silently) that the person feels driven to perform in response to an obsession or according to rigid rules. The goal of the compulsion is to **reduce the anxiety** caused by the obsession or prevent some dreaded event—however, the relief is temporary, and the act is often excessive or not realistically connected to the feared outcome.

OCD is **time-consuming** (often taking >1 hour per day) and causes marked distress or impairment in functioning. Individuals usually recognize their obsessions/compulsions are excessive or unreasonable (though insight can vary).

Nursing Priorities:

1. **Build Trusting Relationship:** Be empathetic and non-judgmental about seemingly bizarre thoughts or behaviors.

2. **Ensure Basic Needs:** Obsessions/compulsions can interfere with eating, sleeping, hygiene. Monitor and assist as needed.

3. **Assess Skin Integrity:** Excessive washing can damage skin. Provide skin care.

4. **Initially, Allow Rituals (unless harmful):** Do *not* interrupt compulsions abruptly at first, as this drastically increases anxiety. Provide for safety and allow completion.

5. **Gradually Set Limits (Collaboratively):** Once rapport is established, work *with* the patient and treatment team to gradually limit the *time* spent on rituals (e.g., "Let's try to limit handwashing to 5 minutes this time"). Provide alternative coping mechanisms.

6. **Therapeutic Communication:** Encourage verbalization of anxieties and triggers for obsessions. Help patient connect obsessions and compulsions.

7. **Medication Education:** SSRIs (often at higher doses than for depression) are first-line treatment. Explain purpose, side effects, importance of adherence.

8. **Support Exposure and Response Prevention (ERP):** This is a specific type of CBT and the gold standard therapy

for OCD. It involves exposing the patient to obsessive triggers while preventing them from engaging in the compulsive ritual. Nurses support patients undergoing ERP, manage anxiety, and reinforce therapist instructions.

9. **Stress Management:** Teach relaxation techniques to manage underlying anxiety.

Case Snippet: OCD

- *Scenario:* Sarah, 35, spends 3-4 hours daily cleaning her kitchen counters with bleach, convinced they are contaminated with deadly germs. She has intrusive thoughts of her family getting sick. She must wash her hands 20 times after touching any surface outside her home. Her hands are red, cracked, and painful. She avoids social outings for fear of contamination.

- *Nursing Considerations:* Priorities for Sarah include assessing skin integrity and providing barrier creams, understanding the specific obsessions (contamination) and compulsions (cleaning/washing), building rapport without judgment, educating her about OCD and treatment options (SSRIs, ERP), collaborating on a plan to gradually limit cleaning time while teaching anxiety management techniques, and ensuring she maintains adequate nutrition/hydration which might be neglected due to time spent on rituals.

What to Watch For (OCD):

- Time consumed by obsessions/compulsions.

- Level of distress caused.

- Physical consequences (skin damage, exhaustion).

- Impact on relationships, work/school functioning.

- Avoidance of triggers.

- Co-occurring conditions (anxiety disorders, depression, tic disorders).

Common Nursing Diagnoses (OCD):

- **Anxiety** (severe)

- **Ineffective Coping**

- **Impaired Skin Integrity**

- **Social Isolation**

- **Fatigue**

- **Risk for Infection** (due to skin breakdown)

Perspectives on Pervasive Worry

Anxiety disorders and OCD illustrate how normal protective mechanisms—like fear, worry, or attention to detail—can become dysregulated, causing profound distress and interfering with life. Nursing care requires patience, empathy, and a focus on practical strategies. We aim not necessarily to eliminate anxiety—a perhaps impossible task—but to help individuals develop the skills and supports needed to manage it effectively, reducing its control over their lives. Understanding the specific patterns of GAD, Panic Disorder, Phobias, and OCD allows us to tailor our approach, always remembering the suffering these conditions inflict and the courage it takes to confront them. Next, we shift our focus to disorders primarily affecting mood: the depressive disorders.

Core Learnings from This Section

- **Anxiety Disorders** involve excessive fear/worry interfering with function.

- **GAD:** Chronic, excessive worry about multiple things + physical symptoms (restlessness, fatigue, muscle tension, etc.). Nurse: Calm approach, coping skills, CBT principles.

- **Panic Disorder:** Recurrent, unexpected panic attacks + fear of future attacks. Nurse (during attack): Stay calm, stay with patient, simple directions, breathing; (between attacks): Education, coping skills. Watch for agoraphobia.

- **Phobias:** Intense, irrational fear of specific object/situation leading to avoidance. Nurse: Acknowledge fear, relaxation, support exposure therapy principles.

- **OCD:** Obsessions (intrusive thoughts/urges) + Compulsions (repetitive behaviors/mental acts to reduce anxiety). Nurse: Allow rituals initially (if safe), gradually limit time, support ERP, manage physical consequences (skin).

- Core nursing priorities across these disorders include **building trust, therapeutic communication, teaching coping/relaxation skills, medication education, and promoting self-care.**

Chapter 7: Depressive Disorders

While everyone feels sad or "blue" occasionally, depressive disorders are different. They involve persistent, pervasive low mood or loss of interest, accompanied by a range of emotional, cognitive, physical, and behavioral symptoms that significantly impair functioning. Depression is not weakness or something one can simply "snap out of." It is a serious medical condition that requires understanding and treatment. As nurses, encountering depression is common—not just in psychiatric settings, but across all areas of healthcare. Recognizing its signs and providing appropriate care, especially ensuring safety, is a fundamental nursing responsibility.

Major Depressive Disorder MDD

Major Depressive Disorder (MDD) is defined by the presence of one or more **Major Depressive Episodes (MDEs)**. An MDE involves a period of at least two weeks during which the person experiences either **depressed mood** or **loss of interest or pleasure (anhedonia)** nearly every day, plus several associated symptoms.

Key Symptoms (SIGECAPS Mnemonic): A useful way to remember the core symptoms of an MDE (need 5 or more, including one of the first two, for diagnosis):

- **S**leep: Insomnia (difficulty falling/staying asleep, early morning awakening) OR hypersomnia (sleeping too much).

- **I**nterest: Markedly diminished interest or pleasure in almost all activities (anhedonia). This is a key symptom.

- **G**uilt: Feelings of worthlessness or excessive/inappropriate guilt (may be delusional).

- **E**nergy: Fatigue or loss of energy nearly every day.

- **C**oncentration: Diminished ability to think or concentrate, or indecisiveness.

- **A**ppetite: Significant weight loss (when not dieting) or weight gain, or decrease/increase in appetite.

- **P**sychomotor: Observable psychomotor agitation (restlessness, pacing, hand-wringing) OR retardation (slowed speech, thought, movement).

- **S**uicidal Ideation: Recurrent thoughts of death (not just fear of dying), recurrent suicidal ideation without a specific plan, or a suicide attempt or specific plan.

These symptoms cause significant distress or impairment in social, occupational, or other important areas of functioning. They[40] are not attributable to substance use or another medical condition.

Nursing Priorities (MDD):

1. **SAFETY FIRST: Suicide Risk Assessment:** This is the **absolute top priority**. Depression is the leading cause of suicide.

   o Assess **ideation** directly ("Are you having thoughts of hurting yourself?").

   o Assess **plan** ("Do you have a plan?").

   o Assess **intent** ("How likely are you to act on these thoughts?").

   o Assess **means** ("Do you have access to [pills, weapons, etc.]?").

   o Assess **history** of past attempts (strong predictor).

- Assess **risk factors** (hopelessness, impulsivity, substance use, recent loss, isolation, severe symptoms).

- Implement **safety precautions** based on risk level (e.g., 1:1 observation, removing dangerous objects, safety contract - though contracts alone are insufficient).

2. **Therapeutic Relationship:** Build trust through empathy, consistency, and non-judgment. Spend time with withdrawn patients, even in silence initially. Convey hope (realistic hope, not false reassurance).

3. **Medication Management:**

- Administer antidepressants as ordered (SSRIs, SNRIs, TCAs, MAOIs, atypicals).

- **Educate** patient/family about:

  - Purpose and mechanism (simplified).

  - Common side effects (and how to manage them).

  - **Therapeutic Lag:** Emphasize that antidepressants take **weeks** (often 2-6) to reach full effect – crucial to prevent premature discontinuation.

  - **Suicide Risk during Early Treatment:** Energy might return *before* mood lifts, potentially increasing suicide risk initially. Monitor closely.

  - Importance of **not stopping abruptly** (discontinuation syndrome).

- Specific precautions (e.g., diet for MAOIs, monitoring for Serotonin Syndrome).

4. **Promote Self-Care (Activities of Daily Living - ADLs):** Depression often causes neglect of hygiene, grooming, nutrition.

   o Encourage (don't force) basic hygiene – offer assistance if needed. Break tasks down (e.g., "Let's just wash your face now").

   o Monitor intake and output. Encourage fluids and nutrition. Offer small, frequent meals if appetite is poor.

   o Structure sleep/wake times. Discourage daytime napping if insomnia is present.

5. **Encourage Activity:** Combat psychomotor retardation and anhedonia.

   o Start small (e.g., sitting out of bed for 15 minutes, a short walk).

   o Gradually increase activity level. Simple exercise can improve mood.

   o Encourage participation in unit activities/groups, even passive involvement initially.

6. **Cognitive Strategies:** Help patients recognize and challenge negative thought patterns (worthlessness, hopelessness, guilt). Encourage focus on small accomplishments. Reinforce strengths.

7. **Provide Structure:** A predictable daily routine can be comforting and help activate the patient.

8. **Patient/Family Education:** Teach about depression as an illness, treatment options, warning signs of relapse.

Case Snippet: MDD

- *Scenario:* Mrs. Davis, 65, is admitted after her daughter found her neglecting herself at home following her husband's death 3 months prior. Mrs. Davis reports feeling "empty" and "useless," has lost 15 pounds, rarely gets out of bed, cries frequently, and expresses thoughts like "There's no point in going on without him." She admits to thinking about taking all her sleeping pills but denies having a specific plan currently.

- *Nursing Considerations:* Highest priority is ongoing suicide risk assessment and ensuring a safe environment. Building rapport is key – sitting with her, acknowledging her grief and pain without minimizing it. Nursing care will focus on monitoring safety (e.g., frequent checks), encouraging nutrition and hygiene (perhaps assisting with meals, offering gentle prompts for bathing), administering antidepressants and monitoring for effects/side effects (especially watching for increased energy before mood lifts), providing opportunities for expressing feelings, and instilling hope by focusing on small steps and potential for improvement with treatment.

What to Watch For (MDD):

- **Suicidal Cues:** Giving away possessions, sudden improvement in mood after deep depression (may indicate decision to act), direct or indirect statements about death/dying/hopelessness.

- **Vegetative Signs:** Significant changes in sleep, appetite, energy, libido – indicate severity.

- **Psychotic Features:** Delusions (often mood-congruent, like guilt or somatic delusions) or hallucinations.

- **Response to Medication:** Both therapeutic effects and side effects.

- **Self-Care Deficits:** Neglect of hygiene, nutrition, environment.

- Social withdrawal.

Persistent Depressive Disorder PDD Dysthymia

Think of **Persistent Depressive Disorder (PDD)**, formerly known as Dysthymia, as a lower-grade but much more **chronic** form of depression. The mood is depressed for most of the day, for more days than not, for **at least two years** (one year for children/adolescents).

Symptoms: While mood is depressed, the associated symptoms are fewer or less intense than in an MDE. Need two or more of the following:

- Poor appetite or overeating.

- Insomnia or hypersomnia.

- Low energy or fatigue.

- Low self-esteem.

- Poor concentration[43] or difficulty making decisions.

- Feelings of hopelessness.

Individuals with PDD haven't been without these symptoms for more than two months at a time during the 2-year period. While perhaps less acutely disabling than MDD day-to-day, its chronicity can significantly wear people down, impacting relationships, work, and overall quality of life. People with PDD may say, "I've always been this way." They are also at higher risk for developing episodes of Major Depressive Disorder on top of their chronic low mood ("double depression").

Nursing Priorities (PDD):

Priorities often overlap with MDD, but with adjustments for chronicity:

1. **Thorough Assessment:** Assess for current MDD symptoms (double depression) and suicide risk (still a concern, though perhaps lower than in acute MDD unless an MDE is superimposed).

2. **Focus on Functioning:** Identify how chronic low mood impacts daily life, relationships, work.

3. **Psychotherapy Emphasis:** Psychotherapy (CBT, interpersonal therapy) is often very helpful for PDD, addressing long-standing patterns of thinking and behaving. Nurses support engagement in therapy.

4. **Medication Education/Adherence:** Antidepressants may be used, often long-term. Education about chronicity and the need for sustained treatment is important.

5. **Instilling Hope:** Help patients recognize that improvement *is* possible, even if the low mood feels "normal" to them. Focus on gradual changes and improved quality of life.

6. **Coping Strategies:** Teach stress management and coping skills suitable for long-term use.

7. **Identify Strengths:** Help patients recognize their resilience in managing chronic symptoms.

Case Snippet: PDD

- *Scenario:* Mark, 30, seeks counseling at his workplace EAP. He describes feeling generally "blah" and pessimistic for as long as he can remember. He enjoys few things, struggles with motivation at work (though manages to keep his job), feels chronically tired, and often criticizes himself harshly. He denies suicidal thoughts but feels life is generally joyless and a struggle. He can't recall ever feeling truly happy for a prolonged period.

- *Nursing Considerations (EAP Counselor/Nurse):* Assessment suggests PDD. Priorities include validating his long-term struggle, psychoeducation about PDD, exploring the impact on his life, strongly recommending psychotherapy (CBT could target negative self-talk and behavioral activation), discussing potential benefits/drawbacks of antidepressant medication with him and referring to a prescriber if interested, and helping him set realistic goals for improving quality of life and identifying small, positive activities.

Suicide Risk Factors Recap A Constant Vigil

Because depression carries such a high risk of suicide, it bears repeating key factors to keep in mind during *any* assessment:

Static Risk Factors (Historical/Unchangeable):

- **Previous Suicide Attempt(s):** Strongest predictor.
- **Family History:** Suicide, mental illness, substance abuse.
- **History of Trauma/Abuse.**
- **Chronic Medical Illness.**
- **Demographics:** (Note: these are statistical, never used alone to judge individual risk) Older males, younger adults, specific ethnic groups can have higher rates.

Dynamic Risk Factors (Modifiable/Current State):

- **Current Mental Disorder:** Especially MDD, Bipolar Disorder, Schizophrenia, Substance Use Disorder, Borderline Personality Disorder, Anxiety Disorders.

- **Suicidal Ideation:** Frequency, intensity, duration.
- **Specific Plan & Intent:** Lethality of plan, preparedness.
- **Hopelessness:** Pervasive belief things won't get better.
- **Anhedonia:** Loss of interest/pleasure.
- **Impulsivity/Poor Judgment.**
- **Agitation/Severe Anxiety/Panic Attacks.**
- **Psychotic Symptoms:** Especially command hallucinations.
- **Substance Abuse/Intoxication.**
- **Recent Loss or Stressor:** Relationship breakup, job loss, financial crisis, death of loved one.
- **Social Isolation/Lack of Support.**
- **Access to Lethal Means.**
- **Recent Discharge from Psychiatric Hospital:** High-risk period.

Protective Factors (Buffers):

- Strong social support/family connection.
- Good coping skills/problem-solving abilities.
- Sense of responsibility (e.g., to children, pets).
- Access to and engagement in effective mental health care.
- Hopefulness/Reasons for living.
- Restricted access to lethal means.
- Cultural/religious beliefs discouraging suicide.

Always ask directly. Assess thoroughly. Document clearly. Implement safety measures. Never assume.

Thoughts on the Weight of Depression

Depression casts a long shadow, draining color and energy from life. It requires immense effort for individuals just to get through the day. As nurses, our role extends far beyond medication passes. It involves bearing witness to suffering without flinching, offering consistent support, ensuring safety above all else, challenging the hopelessness that depression breeds, and holding onto hope *for* the patient until they can reclaim it themselves. It's about promoting small steps toward light—a shower taken, a meal eaten, a moment of connection—recognizing these as significant victories in the face of overwhelming psychic pain. Understanding depression allows us to respond not with judgment, but with the informed compassion and vigilant care these individuals need and deserve. We now turn to conditions where mood swings can climb to euphoric or irritable heights, contrasting sharply with depressive lows: the bipolar disorders.

Core Learnings from This Section

- **Depressive Disorders** involve persistent low mood or anhedonia plus other symptoms impairing function.

- **MDD:** Characterized by Major Depressive Episodes (use **SIGECAPS** mnemonic: Sleep, Interest, Guilt, Energy, Concentration, Appetite, Psychomotor, Suicidality).

- **PDD (Dysthymia):** Chronic, lower-grade depression lasting at least 2 years.

- **Nursing Priority #1 for Depression is SAFETY:** Always conduct thorough suicide risk assessment and implement precautions.

- Other key priorities include **therapeutic relationship, medication management (educate on lag time!), promoting self-care/ADLs, encouraging activity, cognitive strategies, and providing structure/hope.**

- Be aware of **risk factors** and **protective factors** for suicide. Ask directly!

Chapter 8: Bipolar and Related Disorders

Life naturally involves emotional ups and downs. But for individuals with bipolar and related disorders, these shifts are extreme, moving between poles of intense energy, euphoria, or irritability (mania or hypomania) and profound depression. These are not just mood swings; they are episodes of distinct mood states that can severely disrupt thinking, judgment, behavior, and overall functioning. Understanding the different types of bipolar disorder and the characteristics of each mood state is essential for providing safe and effective nursing care, which often involves navigating complex and challenging behaviors.

Mania Versus Hypomania Versus Depression

Recognizing the different mood states is key to understanding bipolar disorders.

- **Manic Episode (Mania):** A distinct period of abnormally and persistently elevated, expansive, or irritable mood, AND persistently increased goal-directed activity or energy, lasting **at least 1 week** (or any duration if hospitalization is necessary). During this period, three or more specific symptoms (four if the mood is only irritable) are present to a significant degree. The mood disturbance is severe enough to cause **marked impairment** in social or occupational functioning, or to **necessitate hospitalization** to prevent harm to self or others, or there are **psychotic features** (delusions, hallucinations). It's a dramatic shift from the person's usual self.

- **Hypomanic Episode (Hypomania):** Similar symptoms to mania (elevated/irritable mood, increased energy/activity) but less severe. The episode lasts **at least 4 consecutive days**. It involves a definite change in

125

functioning that is observable by others, but it is **NOT severe enough** to cause marked impairment in functioning or require hospitalization. There are **NO psychotic features**. While less severe than mania, hypomania is still a distinct change from normal functioning and can lead to problematic decisions or behaviors.

- **Major Depressive Episode (Depression):** This is the same as described in the previous section on Major Depressive Disorder (MDD). Characterized by depressed mood or loss of interest/pleasure (anhedonia) plus other SIGECAPS symptoms for at least 2 weeks, causing significant distress or impairment.

It's the presence and severity of mania or hypomania that differentiate bipolar disorders from MDD.

Bipolar I Versus Bipolar II

The main distinction lies in the severity of the "up" episodes:

- **Bipolar I Disorder:** Defined by the occurrence of **at least one full Manic Episode**. Individuals with Bipolar I *may* also experience hypomanic episodes and major depressive episodes, but the diagnosis only requires the history of a single manic episode. Mania is the defining feature. The highs are very high, often leading to hospitalization or psychosis.

- **Bipolar II Disorder:** Defined by a history of **at least one Hypomanic Episode** AND **at least one Major Depressive Episode**. Individuals with Bipolar II have **NEVER** had a full manic episode. If full mania occurs, the diagnosis changes to Bipolar I. People with Bipolar II often experience longer periods of depression and the hypomania might be less recognized or even feel

126

productive initially, but the depressive episodes cause significant impairment and suffering.

Why the distinction matters: While both are serious, the risks and management can differ. The extreme highs of mania in Bipolar I often lead to more severe consequences (legal issues, financial ruin, relationship damage, need for hospitalization). People with Bipolar II might suffer longer with depression and may be misdiagnosed with MDD if hypomania isn't identified.

Key Symptoms of Mania DIGFAST Mnemonic

During a manic episode (required for Bipolar I), look for elevated/expansive/irritable mood plus increased energy/activity, and three (or four if mood is only irritable) of the following symptoms (use the mnemonic **DIGFAST**):

- **D**istractibility: Attention easily drawn to unimportant or irrelevant external stimuli. Difficulty filtering input.

- **I**ndiscretion/Impulsivity: Excessive involvement in activities with high potential for painful consequences (e.g., unrestrained buying sprees, foolish business investments, sexual indiscretions). Poor judgment.

- **G**randiosity: Inflated self-esteem or grandiosity, ranging from unrealistic self-confidence to delusional beliefs about power, knowledge, or identity.

- **F**light of Ideas/Racing Thoughts: Subjective experience that thoughts are racing; observed as abrupt shifts from one topic to another, speech is often rapid and pressured.

- **A**ctivity Increase: Marked increase in goal-directed activity (socially, at work/school, sexually) or psychomotor agitation (purposeless non-goal-directed activity).

- **Sleep Deficit:** Decreased *need* for sleep (e.g., feels rested after only 3 hours). Different from insomnia where one *wants* to sleep but can't.

- **Talkativeness/Pressured Speech:** More talkative than usual, difficult to interrupt, speech feels driven or pressured.

Nursing Priorities During Mania:

1. **SAFETY FIRST:** This is paramount due to impulsivity and poor judgment.

   o **Protect from Harm:** Prevent risky behaviors (spending, sexual indiscretions, driving recklessly). This may require setting firm limits, close observation, or even seclusion/restraint in emergencies per protocol.

   o **Assess Suicide Risk:** Despite euphoria, risk can be high due to impulsivity, potential for mixed states (mania + depression simultaneously), or crashing into depression after mania.

   o **Maintain Safe Milieu:** Protect other patients from intrusive or provocative behavior.

2. **Physiological Needs:** Often neglected during mania.

   o **Nutrition/Hydration:** Patients may be too "busy" or distracted to eat/drink. Offer frequent, high-calorie, high-protein finger foods and drinks they can consume "on the go." Monitor intake/output.

   o **Sleep/Rest:** Energy seems boundless, but exhaustion occurs. Provide a quiet environment, encourage short rest periods during the day, reduce stimuli (especially at night), administer sleep medication if ordered.

- ○ **Hygiene/ADLs:** Gently remind and assist with basic hygiene, grooming. Break tasks down.

3. **Milieu Management:** Structure and limit setting are key.

    - ○ **Reduce Stimuli:** Provide a quiet environment; limit group activities initially if overwhelming; minimize noise, lights, people.

    - ○ **Set Clear, Firm Limits:** Address intrusive, manipulative, or provocative behaviors consistently and matter-of-factly. All staff should be consistent. Avoid power struggles.

    - ○ **Provide Structure:** A predictable schedule can help contain behavior. Offer appropriate outlets for energy (e.g., walking with staff, simple tasks) but avoid overly stimulating or competitive activities.

4. **Therapeutic Communication:**

    - ○ Use a **calm, firm, matter-of-fact** tone.

    - ○ Keep communication **brief, simple, and concrete.** Avoid abstract ideas.

    - ○ **Redirect** energy and attention from unsafe or inappropriate activities. "Let's walk over here now."

    - ○ **Avoid arguing** or trying to "reason" with grandiose or irritable patients during acute mania. Focus on safety and limits.

    - ○ **Consistency** in approach among all staff members is vital.

5. **Medication Management:** Mood stabilizers (e.g., lithium, valproic acid, carbamazepine, lamotrigine) are the cornerstone. Antipsychotics (often atypical) are frequently used during acute mania for sedation and to target psychosis/agitation.

   o Administer meds as ordered. Monitor effectiveness and side effects (e.g., lithium toxicity requires close monitoring).

   o Provide clear education once the patient is able to process it.

Case Snippet: Mania (Bipolar I)

- *Scenario:* Mr. Lee, 38, diagnosed with Bipolar I Disorder, is admitted involuntarily. He hasn't slept for 4 days, talks constantly in a pressured, rhyming manner (clang associations), jumps from topic to topic (flight of ideas), and believes he has developed a cure for cancer. He is hyperactive, pacing the halls, trying to organize elaborate "business meetings" with other patients, and has spent $10,000 online on unnecessary items in the past week. He is irritable when staff try to redirect him.

- *Nursing Considerations:* Immediate priorities are safety (preventing further spending/risky behavior, protecting others from intrusiveness) and physiological stability (assessing hydration/nutrition, promoting rest). Nursing actions include: maintaining low stimuli, offering finger foods/fluids frequently, attempting brief redirection ("Mr. Lee, let's take a walk down this hallway now"), setting firm limits on intrusive behavior ("Mr. Lee, please step back and allow Mr. Jones some space"), administering mood stabilizers/antipsychotics as ordered, monitoring vital signs and lithium levels (if applicable), ensuring safety through close observation, and communicating concisely/consistently.

Nursing Priorities During Depression (Bipolar Disorder):

These are largely the same as for MDD:

- **Safety:** High suicide risk, especially as bipolar depression can be severe.

- **Physiological Needs:** Address sleep, appetite, energy deficits.

- **Medication:** Mood stabilizers are continued; antidepressants may be added cautiously (risk of inducing mania/hypomania). Education is key.

- **Therapeutic Relationship:** Empathy, support, instilling hope.

- **Promoting Functioning:** Encourage self-care, activity, structure.

Comparing Mania and Depression Text Description

While existing within the same disorder for many individuals, mania and depression present as near opposites in several key areas:

- **Mood:** In **mania**, mood is typically elevated, expansive, euphoric, or sometimes extremely irritable. In **depression**, mood is persistently sad, empty, or hopeless.

- **Activity Level: Mania** involves significantly increased goal-directed activity or psychomotor agitation; the person feels tireless. **Depression** often brings fatigue, loss of energy, and psychomotor retardation or sometimes agitation.

- **Speech: Manic** speech is often rapid, pressured, talkative, and hard to interrupt. **Depressed** speech may be slowed, hesitant, involve poverty of speech, or have a monotonous tone.

- **Thought Processes: Mania** is associated with racing thoughts and flight of ideas. **Depression** often involves slowed thinking, difficulty concentrating, and rumination on negative themes.

- **Thought Content: Mania** frequently includes grandiosity (inflated self-esteem, belief in special powers). **Depression** features themes of worthlessness, guilt, and hopelessness. Both states can involve psychosis (delusions/hallucinations), but the content often differs (grandiose in mania, nihilistic or guilty in depression).

- **Sleep:** A hallmark of **mania** is a *decreased need* for sleep while still feeling energetic. **Depression** typically involves insomnia or hypersomnia, with accompanying fatigue.

- **Behavior: Mania** leads to impulsive, risky, or intrusive behaviors. **Depression** often results in withdrawal, apathy, and neglect of self-care.

Understanding these contrasting presentations helps nurses tailor interventions appropriately depending on the patient's current mood state.

Navigating the Poles

Working with individuals experiencing bipolar disorder requires flexibility and sharp assessment skills. The nurse must constantly gauge the patient's mood state, anticipate potential risks—whether from manic impulsivity or depressive despair—and adjust the approach accordingly. Safety remains the anchor, particularly during the extremes of mania or severe depression. Providing structure, maintaining clear boundaries, managing the milieu effectively, ensuring physiological stability, and administering medications carefully are all critical components of care. It's about helping the individual navigate these turbulent mood shifts while working towards long-term stability and recovery. From the heights of mania, we now turn to disorders where the primary disturbance involves a break from reality itself: the schizophrenia spectrum.

Core Learnings from This Section

- **Bipolar Disorders** involve shifts between mania/hypomania and depression

- **Mania:** Elevated/irritable mood, increased energy, >=1 week, marked impairment/hospitalization/psychosis. Key symptoms: **DIGFAST** (Distractibility, Indiscretion, Grandiosity, Flight of ideas, Activity increase, Sleep deficit, Talkativeness).

- **Hypomania:** Less severe than mania, >=4 days, observable change, NO marked impairment/hospitalization/psychosis

- **Bipolar I:** Requires at least one Manic episode.

- **Bipolar II:** Requires Hypomania AND Depression (no full Mania)

- Nursing priorities in **Mania: SAFETY** (impulsivity, risk), **Physiological needs** (sleep, nutrition), **Milieu** (low stimuli, limits), **Communication** (calm, firm, simple), **Medication** (mood stabilizers, antipsychotics).

- Nursing priorities in **Bipolar Depression:** Similar to MDD (Safety, self-care, meds).

- Mania and Depression present with contrasting symptoms in mood, activity, speech, thought, sleep, and behavior.

Chapter 9:Schizophrenia Spectrum and Other Psychotic Disorders

Schizophrenia and related disorders represent some of the most complex and often misunderstood mental health conditions. Their defining feature is **psychosis**, a state involving a loss of contact with reality, fundamentally altering a person's thoughts, perceptions, feelings, and behavior. These are not "split personalities" (a common misconception), but rather brain disorders that fragment thinking and perception. Care requires immense patience, specialized communication skills, a focus on safety, and long-term support for both the individual and their family.

Positive Versus Negative Symptoms Explained

Symptoms of schizophrenia spectrum disorders are often categorized into two main groups—positive and negative—plus cognitive symptoms. Understanding this distinction helps in assessment and treatment planning.

- **Positive Symptoms:** These represent an **excess or distortion** of normal functions. They are "added" experiences that shouldn't be there. They tend to be more dramatic and are often the reason for initial hospitalization. Examples include:

    o **Hallucinations:** False sensory perceptions (hearing voices, seeing things, etc. - discussed in MSE section). Auditory hallucinations are most common.

    o **Delusions:** Fixed, false beliefs (persecutory, grandiose, somatic, etc. - discussed in MSE section).

- Disorganized Thinking/Speech: Difficulty organizing thoughts logically, reflected in speech patterns (loose associations, tangentiality, incoherence/word salad, clang associations, neologisms - see MSE section). This is a core feature.

- Grossly Disorganized or Catatonic Behavior: Behavior ranging from childlike silliness to unpredictable agitation, or marked decrease in reactivity to the environment (catatonia - immobility, mutism, bizarre postures, etc.).

- **Negative Symptoms:** These represent a **diminution or loss** of normal functions. They are things "missing" that should be present. Negative symptoms are often more persistent, less responsive to older medications, and contribute significantly to poor long-term functioning and quality of life. Examples include:

  - **Affective Flattening (or Blunting):** Reduced intensity of emotional expression; face appears immobile, poor eye contact, monotonous voice.

  - **Alogia:** Poverty of speech (reduced amount of speech) or poverty of content (speech amount is adequate, but vague, repetitive, conveys little information).

  - **Avolition:** Lack of motivation or ability to initiate and persist in goal-directed activities (e.g., work, school, self-care). Apathy.

  - **Anhedonia:** Decreased ability to experience pleasure from positive stimuli or to recall pleasure previously experienced.

- o **Asociality:** Apparent lack of interest in social interactions; withdrawal.

- **Cognitive Symptoms:** These involve problems with information processing, attention, memory, and executive functions (planning, problem-solving, abstract thinking). They are common and strongly linked to functional impairment.

Individuals experience different combinations and severities of these symptoms, which can fluctuate over time.

Delusions Hallucinations Disorganized Thinking Speech

These positive symptoms are often the most striking features of psychosis.

- **Delusions:** As noted, these are fixed, false beliefs resistant to reason. It's crucial *not* to argue about the delusion's reality. Focus instead on the underlying feeling or fear the delusion might represent, and gently orient to reality.

  - o *Example:* Patient: "The CIA implanted a chip in my brain." Nurse: "That must feel frightening, thinking someone could control you like that. I don't know about chips, but let's talk about how you're feeling safe here on the unit." (Validates feeling, presents reality simply, redirects to safety).

- **Hallucinations:** False sensory experiences. Assess type, content (especially command hallucinations urging harm), frequency, intensity, and the patient's response. Help the patient learn coping strategies (reality testing - "I know the voices aren't real," distraction, ignoring, using headphones, talking to someone).

- *Example:* Patient appears distressed, looking around fearfully. Nurse: "You look frightened. Are you hearing the voices now?" Patient: "Yes, they're yelling!" Nurse: "That sounds very upsetting. Let's try [a specific coping technique patient has learned], or would you like to walk and talk with me for a bit?" (Assesses, validates feeling, offers coping/distraction).

- **Disorganized Thinking/Speech:** Reflected in disturbed thought processes (loose associations, tangentiality, etc.). Communication needs to be clear, concrete, and patient. Break down complex information. Ask for clarification gently if needed. Don't pretend to understand if you don't.

  - *Example:* Nurse: "It's time for lunch now." Patient: "Lunch... box... car... far away... stars shine bright..." Nurse: "It sounds like you have many thoughts at once. Right now, it is lunchtime. Let's walk to the dining room together." (Acknowledges disorganized thought simply, focuses on immediate reality/task).

Key Nursing Priorities

Caring for individuals with schizophrenia spectrum disorders requires a holistic, long-term perspective, focusing on safety, symptom management, functioning, and quality of life.

1. **SAFETY:**

   - **Risk Assessment:** Assess for command hallucinations, paranoid delusions leading to potential aggression or self-harm, suicidal ideation (risk is elevated).

- **Safe Environment:** Ensure patient safety and safety of others on the milieu. Monitor for agitation or escalating behavior.

- **Basic Needs:** Ensure adequate nutrition, hydration, sleep, hygiene, which may be neglected due to symptoms.

2. **Therapeutic Relationship & Communication:**

- **Build Trust:** Use a calm, consistent, predictable, non-judgmental approach. Be patient; trust develops slowly.

- **Clear Communication:** Use simple, concrete language. Avoid ambiguity. Give brief, clear directions.

- **Validate Feelings, Not Delusions:** Acknowledge the patient's experience ("That sounds frightening") without confirming the reality of psychotic symptoms ("I don't see the spiders").

- **Reality Orientation:** Gently reinforce reality—person, place, time, situation. Focus on here-and-now activities.

- **Manage Communication Challenges:** Be patient with disorganized speech. Don't interrupt frequently. Let the patient know if you don't understand.

3. **Medication Management:** Antipsychotic medications are essential for managing positive symptoms.

- **Administer/Monitor:** Ensure adherence (may require long-acting injectables if adherence is poor). Monitor for therapeutic effects.

- Manage Side Effects: This is critical for adherence and well-being. Monitor closely for:

  - *Extrapyramidal Symptoms (EPS):* (More common with older/typical antipsychotics) Akathisia (restlessness), dystonia (muscle spasms), parkinsonism (tremor, rigidity), tardive dyskinesia (involuntary movements - potentially irreversible). Use scales like AIMS.

  - *Metabolic Syndrome:* (More common with newer/atypical antipsychotics) Weight gain, high blood sugar, high cholesterol/triglycerides, high blood pressure. Requires regular monitoring of weight, BMI, waist circumference, glucose, lipids.

  - *Other side effects:* Sedation, orthostatic hypotension, anticholinergic effects (dry mouth, constipation), neuroleptic malignant syndrome (NMS - rare but life-threatening).

- Patient/Family Education: Teach about medication purpose, importance of adherence, side effect recognition/management.

4. **Symptom Management & Coping Skills:**

   - Help patients identify triggers for symptom exacerbation (e.g., stress, substance use).

   - Teach coping strategies for hallucinations/delusions (distraction, reality testing, positive self-talk, seeking support).

   - Help manage anxiety related to symptoms.

5. **Promoting Functioning & Quality of Life:** Address negative and cognitive symptoms.

   - **Social Skills Training:** Teach/practice conversational skills, conflict resolution, assertiveness.

   - **ADL Assistance/Prompting:** Encourage/assist with hygiene, grooming, room care. Use simple, step-by-step instructions.

   - **Structured Activities:** Encourage participation in unit groups/activities to provide structure and social interaction.

   - **Cognitive Enhancement Strategies:** Simple memory aids, routines.

6. **Family Support and Education:** Families are crucial partners. Provide education about the illness, treatment, coping strategies, realistic expectations, and caregiver support resources. Address family burden and stigma.

Case Snippet: Schizophrenia

- *Scenario:* Ben, 22, diagnosed with schizophrenia, is hospitalized due to worsening auditory hallucinations ("voices telling me I'm evil") and paranoid delusions ("my family is trying to poison my food"). He appears disheveled, speaks tangentially, and isolates himself in his room, refusing meals. His affect is flat.

- *Nursing Considerations:* Priorities include ensuring safety (suicide risk assessment due to distressing hallucinations/delusions, monitoring food/fluid intake), building rapport through brief, frequent, non-demanding contacts, administering antipsychotic medication and monitoring for effects/side effects, addressing meal refusal (offering sealed/packaged foods initially to address poison fears, staying with him during meals), communicating clearly and simply, gently orienting to reality ("Ben, I am your nurse, I work at this hospital. The kitchen staff prepared this food."), involving him in simple, structured activities when able, and coordinating with the treatment team and family regarding discharge planning and adherence support.

Tips for Communicating with Patients Experiencing Psychosis (Summary):

- Be calm, patient, respectful.

- Use clear, simple, concrete words. Short sentences.

- Validate distressing *feelings*, not the specific *content* of delusions/hallucinations.

- Gently present reality; don't argue.

- Focus on the here and now.

- Reduce environmental stimuli.

- Be consistent in approach.

- Let them know if you don't understand their speech; ask for clarification simply.

- Assess and address safety concerns proactively.

Symptom Definitions in Brief Text Description

- **Positive Symptoms (Excess/Distortion):**

  - *Hallucinations:* False sensory perceptions without external stimuli.

  - *Delusions:* Fixed, false beliefs resistant to evidence.

o *Disorganized Thinking/Speech:* Impaired logical thought process seen in speech (e.g., loose associations).

o *Disorganized Behavior:* Actions inappropriate to context, catatonia.

- **Negative Symptoms (Loss/Deficit):**

  o *Affective Flattening:* Reduced emotional expression.

  o *Alogia:* Reduced speech output or content.

  o *Avolition:* Decreased motivation/initiation of activity.

  o *Anhedonia:* Decreased ability to experience pleasure.

  o *Asociality:* Decreased interest in social interaction.

Seeing Beyond the Symptoms

Schizophrenia spectrum disorders challenge our understanding of reality itself. The symptoms—hallucinations, delusions, disorganized thoughts—can be profoundly distressing and isolating for the individual experiencing them. Nursing care demands not only clinical skills in managing medications and ensuring safety but also a deep capacity for empathy and persistence in building trust across the divide created by psychosis. By focusing on the person behind the symptoms, addressing their basic needs, helping them manage distressing experiences, supporting medication adherence, and fostering hope for improved functioning and quality of life, nurses play an indispensable role in the long-term journey of recovery.

Core Learnings from This Section

- **Schizophrenia Spectrum Disorders** involve psychosis (loss of contact with reality).

- **Positive Symptoms** are an excess/distortion (hallucinations, delusions, disorganization).

- **Negative Symptoms** are a loss/deficit (flat affect, alogia, avolition, anhedonia, asociality) and impact functioning significantly.

- **Cognitive Symptoms** (attention, memory, executive function) are also common.

- **Key Nursing Priorities: SAFETY** (risk assessment, basic needs), **Therapeutic Relationship/Communication** (trust, clarity, validate feelings not content), **Medication Management** (antipsychotics, adherence, side effect monitoring - EPS, metabolic syndrome), **Symptom Management/Coping Skills**, Promoting **Functioning/Quality of Life**, and **Family Support**.

- Communicate calmly, clearly, concretely; don't argue with psychotic symptoms but gently orient to reality.

Chapter 10: Personality Disorders

We all have a personality—our unique and relatively consistent way of thinking, feeling, and behaving as we interact with the world. Personality *traits* are specific characteristics, like being outgoing, cautious, or conscientious. Most people have a flexible range of traits they adapt to different situations. However, when these patterns become **rigid, inflexible, pervasive across situations**, and lead to **significant distress or impairment** in social, occupational, or personal functioning, we may be looking at a **Personality Disorder**. These aren't temporary states; they are enduring patterns, typically recognizable by adolescence or early adulthood, that deviate markedly from cultural expectations. Working with individuals with personality disorders can be challenging, requiring particular attention to consistency and boundaries.

Understanding Personality Traits Versus Disorders

Think of personality traits existing on a spectrum. Someone might be described as meticulous (a trait), but this only becomes part of Obsessive-Compulsive *Personality Disorder* if that need for orderliness is so extreme and inflexible that it interferes with efficiency, relationships, and overall functioning. Someone might be sensitive to criticism (a trait), but this differs from the pervasive fear of rejection and social inhibition seen in Avoidant Personality Disorder.

The key distinctions for a **Personality Disorder** are:

- **Enduring Pattern:** Long-standing, not just a reaction to a recent stressor.

- **Inflexible & Pervasive:** The patterns show up across a broad range of personal and social situations, not just one area of life.

- **Clinically Significant Distress or Impairment:** Causes problems for the individual (though insight may be limited) or those around them in important areas like work, school, or relationships.

- **Stable & Long Duration:** Onset traced back at least to adolescence or early adulthood.

- **Not Better Explained By:** Another mental disorder, substance use, or a medical condition.

Individuals with personality disorders often struggle with self-identity, self-direction, empathy, and intimacy. Their ways of perceiving the world, managing emotions, and interacting with others are persistently problematic.

Brief Overview of Clusters

Personality disorders are traditionally grouped into three clusters based on descriptive similarities. This isn't a perfect system, but it provides a basic organizational framework.

- **Cluster A: The Odd or Eccentric Cluster**

  - Characterized by behaviors that appear odd, eccentric, or withdrawn.

  - **Paranoid Personality Disorder:** Pervasive distrust and suspiciousness of others, interpreting motives as malevolent. Expects exploitation, questions loyalty, reads hidden threats into benign remarks.

  - **Schizoid Personality Disorder:** Pervasive pattern of detachment from social relationships and a restricted range of emotional[13] expression. Prefers solitary activities, lacks close friends, seems indifferent to praise or criticism.

- o **Schizotypal Personality Disorder:** Pervasive pattern of social and interpersonal deficits marked by acute discomfort with close relationships, plus cognitive or perceptual distortions and eccentricities of behavior. Ideas of reference, odd beliefs/magical thinking, unusual perceptual experiences, odd thinking/speech,[17] suspiciousness, inappropriate affect. (Sometimes considered related to schizophrenia spectrum).

- **Cluster B: The Dramatic, Emotional, or Erratic Cluster**

  - o Characterized by behaviors that appear dramatic, emotional, impulsive, or erratic. Individuals in this cluster often present significant challenges in clinical settings.

  - o **Antisocial Personality Disorder (ASPD):** Pervasive pattern of disregard for and violation of the rights of others. Deceitfulness, impulsivity, irritability/aggressiveness, irresponsibility, lack of remorse. Must be at least 18, with evidence of Conduct Disorder before age 15.

  - o **Borderline Personality Disorder (BPD):** Pervasive pattern of instability in interpersonal relationships, self-image, and affects, along with marked impulsivity. Frantic efforts to avoid abandonment, unstable/intense relationships (idealization/devaluation), identity disturbance, impulsivity[23] (spending, sex, substances, binge eating), recurrent suicidal behavior/gestures/threats or self-mutilation, affective instability (intense mood swings), chronic feelings of emptiness, inappropriate intense anger, transient stress-related paranoia or dissociation.

- o **Histrionic Personality Disorder:** Pervasive pattern of excessive emotionality and attention-seeking. Needs to be center of attention, uses physical appearance to draw attention, rapidly shifting/shallow emotions, considers relationships more intimate than they are, easily suggestible.

- o **Narcissistic Personality Disorder:** Pervasive pattern of grandiosity (in fantasy or behavior), need for admiration, and lack of empathy. Sense of self-importance, preoccupied with fantasies of success/power, believes they are "special," requires excessive admiration, sense of entitlement, interpersonally exploitative, lacks empathy, often envious, arrogant.

- **Cluster C: The Anxious or Fearful Cluster**

  - o Characterized by behaviors that appear anxious or fearful.

  - o **Avoidant Personality Disorder:** Pervasive pattern of social inhibition, feelings of inadequacy, and hypersensitivity[31] to negative evaluation. Avoids occupational activities with interpersonal contact, unwilling to get involved unless certain of being liked, fears criticism/rejection in social situations, views self as socially inept or inferior.

  - o **Dependent Personality Disorder:** Pervasive and excessive need to be taken care of that leads to submissive and clinging behavior and fears of separation. Difficulty making decisions without advice/reassurance, needs others to assume responsibility, fears disagreeing, difficulty initiating projects, goes to excessive lengths for nurturance/support, feels helpless when alone.

- ○ **Obsessive-Compulsive Personality Disorder (OCPD):** Pervasive pattern of preoccupation with orderliness, perfectionism, and mental/interpersonal control, at the expense of flexibility, openness, and efficiency. Preoccupied with details/rules/lists, perfectionism interferes with task completion, excessively devoted to work, inflexible about morality/ethics/values,[40] unable to discard worn-out objects, reluctant to delegate, miserly spending style, rigid and stubborn. **Note:** This is different from OCD; OCPD lacks the true obsessions/compulsions driven by anxiety seen in OCD. It's a pervasive personality style.

Focus on Key Examples Common Challenges for Nurses

While nurses may encounter individuals with any personality disorder, those in Cluster B—particularly Borderline Personality Disorder and Antisocial Personality Disorder—often present unique and significant challenges in healthcare settings due to their impact on relationships and behavior.

Borderline Personality Disorder (BPD):

- **Core Feature:** Instability – in relationships, self-image, mood, and behavior. Intense fear of abandonment drives much of the behavior.

- **Common Presentation:** May present with intense emotional pain, chronic feelings of emptiness, rapid mood shifts (within hours), difficulty controlling anger, impulsive behaviors (self-harm like cutting, burning; suicide attempts; substance use; reckless driving; binge eating), chaotic interpersonal relationships characterized by **splitting** (seeing others as "all good" or "all bad," rapidly shifting between idealizing and devaluing the same person). They may also experience transient paranoid thoughts or dissociative symptoms under stress. Self-harm is often used to cope with intense emotional pain or feelings of emptiness, not necessarily with suicidal intent, but suicide risk is very high.

- **Key Challenges for Nurses:**

  - **Emotional Intensity:** Patient's distress can be overwhelming for staff. Requires maintaining professional calm.

  - **Splitting:** Patient may idealize one staff member ("You're the only one who understands me") while devaluing another ("That other nurse is useless/mean"). This can divide the staff team.

  - **Impulsivity/Self-Harm:** Requires constant safety assessment and management. Need clear protocols for managing self-harm behaviors without reinforcing them.

  - **Boundary Testing:** Patients may push limits to test relationships or seek reassurance.

  - **Countertransference:** Staff may have strong emotional reactions (frustration, anger, pity, desire to rescue) that interfere with therapeutic care. Supervision is essential.

- **Treatment Note:** Dialectical Behavior Therapy (DBT) is a highly effective treatment developed specifically for BPD, focusing on skills for mindfulness, distress tolerance, emotion regulation, and interpersonal effectiveness. Nurses can support DBT principles on the unit.

Case Snippet: BPD

- *Scenario:* Lisa, 22, admitted after cutting her arms superficially following an argument with her boyfriend whom she feared was leaving her. On the unit, she initially praises Nurse A effusively ("You're amazing, so much better than Nurse B"). Later, when Nurse A enforces a unit rule, Lisa becomes intensely angry, yells, calls Nurse A "useless," and demands to speak only with Nurse B, whom she now idealizes. She reports feeling empty and makes vague threats of further self-harm if her boyfriend doesn't call.

- *Nursing Considerations:* Priorities include safety (assessing self-harm risk, securing sharp objects), managing splitting (Nurse A and B must communicate closely, present a united front, avoid taking sides, perhaps Nurse B redirects Lisa back to Nurse A to resolve the conflict), setting firm boundaries on verbal aggression, validating her underlying fear of abandonment without excusing the behavior ("It sounds like you were very scared about your boyfriend, and it's hard when rules feel restrictive, but yelling is not acceptable here"), and encouraging use of coping skills (like distress tolerance skills from DBT, if known).

Antisocial Personality Disorder (ASPD):

- **Core Feature:** Disregard for others' rights, lack of empathy/remorse, often manipulative and deceitful. Focus is on personal gain or pleasure, regardless of consequences for others.

- **Common Presentation:** May appear charming or glib superficially but exploit others. History often includes impulsivity, aggression, irresponsibility (work, finances), lying, and unlawful behavior. They may rationalize their actions or blame victims. Substance use disorders are very common. They rarely seek treatment for ASPD itself but may enter the healthcare system due to legal issues, substance use complications, or feigning illness for secondary gain (e.g., seeking medication).

- **Key Challenges for Nurses:**

  - **Manipulation:** Patients may attempt to manipulate staff for privileges, medications, or to bend rules.

  - **Deceitfulness:** Difficult to trust patient self-report. Need to verify information when possible.

  - **Lack of Empathy/Remorse:** Can be difficult for staff to connect with or feel empathy *for* the patient.

  - **Impulsivity/Aggression:** Potential for rule-breaking, irritability, and aggression towards staff or other patients.

  - **Splitting/Staff Division:** May attempt to pit staff against each other.

  - **Boundary Violations:** May test limits, flatter staff, or attempt inappropriate familiarity.

- **Treatment Note:** Treatment is challenging. Focus is often on managing co-occurring conditions (substance use), addressing specific behaviors (aggression), and setting firm limits within a structured environment (like forensic settings). Building motivation for change is difficult due to lack of insight/remorse.

Case Snippet: ASPD

- *Scenario:* Mr. Jones, 35, is admitted to a detox unit for alcohol withdrawal. He has a long history of arrests for theft and assault. He is initially charming to the female nurses, flattering them while complaining about the male staff being "unfair." He repeatedly requests higher doses of benzodiazepines than his withdrawal score indicates, claiming severe symptoms contradicted by his vital signs and observed behavior. He tries to convince another patient to sneak him cigarettes against unit rules. When confronted about rule-breaking, he becomes verbally abusive and blames staff for "making" him act out.

- *Nursing Considerations:* Priorities include safe management of alcohol withdrawal (using objective tools like CIWA-Ar, administering medication based on scores/vitals, not just subjective complaints), maintaining strict boundaries regarding medication requests and unit rules, ensuring staff consistency in approach (all staff enforce rules equally), managing manipulative behavior matter-of-factly without engaging in power struggles, documenting behavior objectively, ensuring safety of staff and other patients (monitoring for potential aggression), and recognizing that genuine therapeutic rapport may be limited. Focus on the immediate task: safe detox.

Nursing Priorities General Approaches

While each personality disorder is unique, some general nursing principles are particularly helpful, especially when dealing with Cluster B presentations:

1. **Consistency:** All staff members must be on the same page regarding rules, expectations, consequences, and the overall care plan. A consistent approach minimizes

opportunities for splitting and manipulation. Frequent staff communication is key.

2. **Boundary Setting:** This is non-negotiable. Boundaries must be:

   o **Clear:** State the limit directly and simply.

   o **Firm:** Do not waver or negotiate the limit once set.

   o **Consistent:** Apply the limit every time the behavior occurs, by all staff.

   o **Non-Punitive:** State limits matter-of-factly, focusing on safety and therapeutic environment, not punishment.

   o **State Consequences:** Explain what will happen if the limit is not respected (e.g., "If you continue yelling, I will need to end this conversation now and return in 15 minutes when things are calmer").

3. **Managing Splitting:**

   o **Recognize it:** Understand it as a defense mechanism related to difficulty seeing others as having both good and bad qualities.

   o **Avoid Taking Sides:** Do not get drawn into "good nurse/bad nurse" dynamics.

   o **Promote Staff Communication:** Share information about patient interactions and attempts to split staff.

   o **Encourage Direct Communication:** Gently encourage the patient to speak directly to the staff member they have an issue with (if appropriate and safe).

- o **Present United Front:** Reinforce that all staff work together as a team.

4. **Safety:** Continuously assess risk for self-harm, suicide (especially BPD), and aggression/violence towards others (especially ASPD). Implement appropriate safety measures.

5. **Therapeutic Communication:**

- o Maintain a **calm, neutral, matter-of-fact** tone, especially when setting limits or dealing with intense emotions.

- o **Focus on Behaviors:** Discuss specific, observable behaviors rather than making judgments about character ("Yelling is disruptive" vs. "You are being manipulative").

- o **Validate Feelings (where appropriate):** Acknowledge the emotion behind the behavior without condoning the behavior itself ("It sounds like you felt very angry, and yelling is how you expressed it. Let's find other ways to express anger.").

- o **Avoid Power Struggles:** Do not get drawn into arguments. State limits and withdraw if necessary.

6. **Focus on Strengths and Coping:** Help patients identify existing strengths and develop healthier coping mechanisms for managing intense emotions, interpersonal conflict, and impulsivity. Reinforce positive behaviors.

7. **Self-Awareness and Supervision:** Nurses *must* be aware of their own emotional reactions (countertransference) when working with these patients. Frustration, anger, feeling manipulated, or wanting to rescue are common. Regular supervision or consultation with experienced colleagues is essential to maintain objectivity and therapeutic effectiveness.

Boundary Setting Tips Quick Reference

- **Be Prepared:** Anticipate that boundaries will likely be tested.

- **Be Clear & Direct:** Use simple language. "It is not acceptable for you to..."

- **Use "I" Statements (for impact on milieu/care):** "I cannot continue this conversation if you are yelling, as it makes it difficult for us to work together."

- **State the Limit, Not a Request:** "You need to stop yelling now," not "Could you please stop yelling?"

- **Be Consistent:** Apply the limit every time, by everyone.

- **State the Consequence (briefly, calmly):** "If you continue [behavior], then [consequence - e.g., conversation ends, privilege restricted]."

- **Avoid Arguing or Justifying:** State the limit and consequence, then disengage from debate.

- **Remain Calm & Professional:** Even if the patient escalates.

A Note on Navigating Patterns

Working with individuals whose core patterns of relating cause them and others pain requires a unique blend of firmness and empathy. Personality disorders are deeply ingrained, and change is often slow and difficult. Nurses provide care often during crises (hospitalizations, detox) rather than long-term therapy. Our role in these acute settings focuses heavily on managing behavior, ensuring safety, maintaining a therapeutic milieu through consistency and boundaries, and attempting to build enough rapport to address immediate needs. Recognizing the patterns, understanding the underlying dynamics (like fear of abandonment in BPD or lack of remorse in ASPD), and managing our own reactions are fundamental to providing ethical and effective care without burnout. Next, we examine another set of conditions frequently encountered across healthcare settings, often intertwined with other mental health issues: substance use disorders.

Core Learnings from This Section

- **Personality Disorders:** Enduring, inflexible, pervasive patterns of inner experience/behavior causing distress/impairment. Different from flexible personality traits.

- **Three Clusters:** A (Odd/Eccentric), B (Dramatic/Emotional/Erratic), C (Anxious/Fearful).

- **Cluster B (BPD, ASPD)** often present challenges due to instability, impulsivity, manipulation, disregard for others.

- **BPD Key Features:** Instability (relationships, self-image, mood), impulsivity, fear of abandonment, splitting, self-harm.

- **ASPD Key Features:** Disregard/violation of others' rights, deceitfulness, lack of remorse.

- **Nursing Priorities: Consistency** across staff, firm **Boundary Setting**, managing **Splitting**, ensuring **Safety** (self-harm/aggression), using matter-of-fact **Communication**, focusing on **Coping Skills**, and **Nurse Self-Awareness/Supervision** (countertransference).

Chapter 11: Substance Use and Addictive Disorders

Substance use touches nearly every aspect of healthcare. Whether on a medical floor, in the emergency department, a community clinic, or a psychiatric unit, you will care for individuals whose lives are affected by the use—and often misuse—of alcohol, prescription drugs, or illicit substances. Understanding substance use disorders (SUDs) not as moral failings but as complex, chronic brain conditions is essential for providing non-judgmental, effective nursing care. This involves recognizing patterns of intoxication and withdrawal, understanding the interplay with other mental health conditions, and prioritizing safety and supportive interventions.

Commonly Abused Substances Overview

Many substances can be misused, leading to dependence and addiction. Here's a brief look at major categories:

- **Alcohol:** A central nervous system depressant. Chronic heavy use carries significant risks: liver disease (cirrhosis), pancreatitis, cardiovascular problems, brain damage (Wernicke-Korsakoff syndrome), increased cancer risk. **Withdrawal can be life-threatening** (seizures, delirium tremens - DTs).

- **Opioids:** Includes illegal drugs like heroin and fentanyl, as well as prescription pain relievers (oxycodone, hydrocodone, morphine). Cause euphoria, pain relief, sedation. High overdose risk due to **respiratory depression**, especially with potent synthetic opioids like fentanyl. Withdrawal is intensely uncomfortable but usually not medically dangerous on its own (though complications can arise). Medication-Assisted Treatment (MAT) with methadone, buprenorphine, or naltrexone is a key treatment approach.

- **Stimulants:** Includes cocaine, amphetamines, and methamphetamine ("meth"). Cause euphoria, increased energy/alertness, decreased appetite. Risks include heart attack, stroke, seizures, severe dental problems ("meth mouth"), psychosis (paranoia, hallucinations). Withdrawal involves a "crash" with fatigue, depression, increased appetite, intense cravings.

- **Sedatives, Hypnotics, and Anxiolytics:** Primarily benzodiazepines (e.g., diazepam, lorazepam, alprazolam) and barbiturates (less common now). Prescribed for anxiety/insomnia but have high potential for dependence. Overdose risk, especially when combined with alcohol or opioids. **Withdrawal, like alcohol, can be life-threatening** (seizures, delirium). Requires gradual tapering.

- **Cannabis (Marijuana):** Effects vary—relaxation, mild euphoria, altered perception. Risks include potential for dependence (Cannabis Use Disorder), impact on cognitive function (especially in adolescents), possible link to psychosis in vulnerable individuals. Withdrawal symptoms can include irritability, anxiety, sleep disturbance, decreased appetite.

- **Hallucinogens:** LSD, psilocybin ("magic mushrooms"), PCP, ketamine. Cause profound alterations in perception, thought, and mood. Effects are unpredictable ("bad trips"). PCP can cause agitation/violence. Long-term effects less understood, but Hallucinogen Persisting Perception Disorder (HPPD - "flashbacks") can occur.

- **Inhalants:** Solvents, aerosols, gases (e.g., glue, paint thinner, nitrous oxide). Primarily used by adolescents. Extremely dangerous, causing rapid intoxication but can lead to sudden death ("sudden sniffing death"), brain damage, organ damage.

Intoxication Versus Withdrawal Concepts

Understanding these two states is fundamental to nursing care.

- **Intoxication:** This refers to the **direct effects** of the substance on the central nervous system shortly after use. It produces a reversible, substance-specific syndrome involving behavioral and psychological changes (e.g., euphoria, impaired judgment, slurred speech with alcohol; agitation, paranoia with stimulants; sedation, pinpoint pupils with opioids). Nursing care during intoxication focuses on:

  - **Safety:** Preventing falls, accidents, risky behaviors. Monitoring level of consciousness, vital signs (especially respiratory status with opioids/sedatives). Assessing for overdose.

  - **Supportive Care:** Providing a safe environment, reducing stimuli if agitated, offering reassurance.

- **Withdrawal:** This occurs when a person who has developed physiological dependence stops or reduces their use of the substance. The body reacts to the absence of the substance, causing a specific cluster of signs and symptoms, often the *opposite* of the drug's effects (e.g., anxiety, tremors, insomnia during alcohol withdrawal; muscle aches, nausea, diarrhea during opioid withdrawal; fatigue, depression during stimulant withdrawal). Nursing care during withdrawal focuses on:

  - **Safety:** Monitoring for and managing potentially life-threatening withdrawal syndromes (alcohol, benzodiazepines). Seizure precautions, delirium management. Assessing suicide risk (can increase during withdrawal).

- **Symptom Management:** Using standardized assessment tools (like CIWA-Ar, COWS) to gauge severity and guide administration of medications to alleviate symptoms (e.g., benzodiazepines for alcohol withdrawal, comfort meds for opioid withdrawal).

- **Supportive Care:** Providing comfort measures, ensuring hydration/nutrition, promoting rest, offering emotional support and reassurance.

Withdrawal Symptom Highlights (Text Description):

- **Alcohol Withdrawal:** Symptoms typically begin 6-24 hours after last drink, peak at 24-48 hours, can last days. Early signs: anxiety, insomnia, tremors, sweating, palpitations, GI upset. Can progress to **withdrawal seizures** (usually within 12-48 hours) or **delirium tremens (DTs)** (peaks 48-72 hours) - characterized by confusion, disorientation, hallucinations (often visual/tactile), agitation, fever, tachycardia, hypertension. DTs are a medical emergency with significant mortality risk. **CIWA-Ar (Clinical Institute Withdrawal Assessment for Alcohol, revised)** is commonly used to score symptoms (nausea/vomiting, tremor, sweats, anxiety, agitation, tactile/auditory/visual disturbances, headache, orientation) and guide benzodiazepine dosing.

- **Opioid Withdrawal:** Symptoms resemble a severe flu: nausea, vomiting, diarrhea, muscle aches, lacrimation (tearing), rhinorrhea (runny nose), pupillary dilation, piloerection ("goosebumps"), sweating, yawning, fever, insomnia, restlessness, intense cravings. While extremely uncomfortable, typically not life-threatening unless co-occurring medical issues exist. **COWS (Clinical Opiate Withdrawal Scale)** assesses pulse, sweating,

restlessness, pupil size, bone/joint aches, runny
nose/tearing, GI upset, tremor, yawning,
anxiety/irritability to guide supportive treatment.

Basics of Co occurring Disorders Dual Diagnosis

It is extremely common for individuals with SUDs to also have
other mental health disorders, and vice versa. This is often
referred to as **co-occurring disorders** or **dual diagnosis**.

- **Why do they co-occur?**
    - **Self-Medication:** People might use substances to
      cope with symptoms of untreated mental illness
      (e.g., alcohol for social anxiety, stimulants for
      depression).

    - **Substance Use Triggering Mental Illness:** Heavy
      substance use can sometimes trigger or worsen
      underlying vulnerabilities for mental disorders
      (e.g., cannabis and psychosis risk, stimulants and
      mania).

    - **Shared Risk Factors:** Genetics, trauma,
      environmental stress can increase risk for both
      SUDs and other mental illnesses.

Implications for Care:

- **Integrated Treatment is Best:** Treating both the SUD and
  the other mental illness concurrently, ideally by the
  same team or through close collaboration, leads to
  better outcomes than treating them separately or
  sequentially.

- **Complex Presentations:** Symptoms can overlap or mimic
  each other, making diagnosis challenging.
  Intoxication/withdrawal can worsen psychiatric
  symptoms.

- **Treatment Challenges:** Patients may have poorer treatment adherence, higher relapse rates, increased risk of homelessness, hospitalization, and suicide compared to those with only one disorder.

Nursing Role:

- **Thorough Assessment:** Screen for both substance use and other mental health symptoms in all patients. Ask about specific substances, patterns of use, and withdrawal history.

- **Understand Interactions:** Be aware of how substance use affects mental health symptoms and vice versa.

- **Support Integrated Care:** Facilitate communication between mental health and substance abuse treatment providers if separate. Advocate for integrated approaches.

- **Tailor Interventions:** Recognize that standard mental health interventions may need modification for patients with active SUDs.

Nursing Priorities Substance Use Disorders

Caring for individuals with SUDs requires a blend of medical management (especially during withdrawal), psychosocial support, and a non-judgmental, hopeful approach.

1. **Safety:** This is always paramount.

    - **Overdose Management:** Recognize signs, administer naloxone for opioid overdose per protocol, manage respiratory status.

    - **Withdrawal Safety:** Implement protocols for managing potentially dangerous withdrawal (alcohol, sedatives). Use assessment tools (CIWA-

Ar, COWS). Seizure/delirium precautions. Monitor vital signs frequently.

- o **Risk Assessment:** Assess for suicide risk (high during intoxication, withdrawal, and active addiction). Assess for potential violence if intoxicated with certain substances (PCP, stimulants). Provide a safe environment.

2. **Withdrawal Management:**

- o **Systematic Assessment:** Use standardized tools reliably.

- o **Medication Administration:** Administer withdrawal medications (benzodiazepines, comfort meds, MAT) as ordered, monitor effectiveness and side effects.

- o **Supportive Care:** Manage physical symptoms (antiemetics, fluids, rest). Provide comfort measures.

3. **Build Therapeutic Alliance:**

- o **Non-Judgmental Approach:** View addiction as a chronic illness, not a moral failure. Use person-first language ("person with substance use disorder," not "addict" or "alcoholic").

- o **Empathy & Respect:** Understand the challenges of addiction and recovery. Treat patients with dignity.

- o **Motivational Interviewing (MI):** Use MI principles (expressing empathy, developing discrepancy, rolling with resistance, supporting self-efficacy) to help patients explore their ambivalence about change and enhance motivation for treatment. Avoid confrontation.

4. **Education:**

   o **Disease Concept:** Explain addiction as a brain disease.

   o **Effects of Substances:** Provide factual information about risks.

   o **Withdrawal & Treatment:** Explain the process, medication options (including MAT), therapy, support groups (AA, NA, SMART Recovery).

   o **Relapse Prevention:** Discuss triggers, cravings, coping strategies. Frame relapse as a potential part of recovery, not a failure.

5. **Promote Healthy Coping:** Help patients identify alternatives to substance use for managing stress, difficult emotions, or mental health symptoms. Teach relaxation, stress management.

6. **Harm Reduction:** For patients not ready or able to achieve abstinence, provide education and resources to reduce the negative consequences of ongoing use.

   o *Examples:* Safe injection practices, needle exchange programs, naloxone kits and training for overdose reversal, safer sex education, moderation management strategies (for alcohol, where appropriate), advising against mixing specific substances. Harm reduction acknowledges the reality of ongoing use for some and prioritizes saving lives and reducing harm.

7. **Address Co-occurring Disorders:** Screen for and support treatment of other mental health conditions.

8. **Discharge Planning & Referrals:** Connect patients with appropriate follow-up care (detox, inpatient/outpatient rehab, MAT providers, therapists, support groups, housing resources).

Case Snippet: Alcohol Withdrawal

- *Scenario:* Mr. Smith, 55, admitted to the medical floor for pneumonia, has a history of heavy daily alcohol use (a pint of vodka/day). On hospital day 2, he becomes increasingly tremulous, sweaty, anxious, and reports nausea. His heart rate and blood pressure are elevated.

- *Nursing Considerations:* Recognize these as early signs of alcohol withdrawal. Priority is safe management. Initiate CIWA-Ar scoring protocol immediately. Notify provider. Administer benzodiazepines (e.g., lorazepam) based on CIWA score per order. Implement seizure precautions. Monitor vital signs and CIWA scores frequently (e.g., every 1-4 hours depending on severity). Ensure hydration. Provide reassurance and orientation. Assess for hallucinations or confusion indicating progression towards DTs.

A Perspective on Substance Use Care

Substance use disorders are complex conditions often layered with stigma, shame, and co-occurring mental health challenges. Effective nursing care demands a shift from judgment to compassion, from confrontation to collaboration. Prioritizing safety during intoxication and withdrawal is essential medical care. Beyond that, building trust, providing education, supporting motivation for change (using approaches like

Motivational Interviewing), teaching coping skills, and embracing harm reduction strategies when appropriate are key elements. Recovery is a long-term process, often involving setbacks, but nurses play a critical role in supporting individuals at every stage of their journey. From the physiological crises of withdrawal, we now turn to conditions born from overwhelming stress and trauma.

Core Learnings from This Section

- **Substance Use Disorders (SUDs)** are chronic brain diseases, not moral failures.

- **Intoxication** involves direct substance effects; **Withdrawal** occurs upon cessation/reduction in dependent individuals. Withdrawal from alcohol/sedatives can be life-threatening.

- **Co-occurring Disorders** (SUD + other mental illness) are common and require integrated treatment.

- **Nursing Priorities: SAFETY** (overdose, withdrawal complications, suicide risk), **Withdrawal Management** (using tools like CIWA-Ar, COWS, administering meds), **Therapeutic Alliance** (non-judgmental, MI principles), **Education** (disease concept, treatment, relapse prevention), promoting **Coping Skills**, and understanding **Harm Reduction**.

- Be familiar with common substances, their effects, and withdrawal patterns (esp. alcohol, opioids, sedatives, stimulants).

Chapter 12: Trauma Stressor Related and Dissociative Disorders

Life inevitably brings stress, but sometimes events are so overwhelming—so terrifying, horrific, or violating—that they leave deep psychological wounds. Trauma- and Stressor-Related Disorders, like Post-Traumatic Stress Disorder (PTSD) and Acute Stress Disorder (ASD), are conditions directly linked to experiencing or witnessing such events. Dissociative disorders also often have roots in trauma, involving disruptions in consciousness, memory, or identity as a way of coping. Understanding the impact of trauma is crucial for nurses in all settings, guiding us towards a more sensitive and effective approach known as Trauma-Informed Care.

Post Traumatic Stress Disorder PTSD

Post-Traumatic Stress Disorder (PTSD) can develop after exposure to actual or threatened death, serious injury, or sexual violence. Exposure can be direct (experiencing it yourself), witnessed (seeing it happen to others), learned (event happened to close family/friend), or through repeated/extreme exposure to aversive details (e.g., first responders). The key is the *response* to the trauma, which persists long after the event and involves distinct symptom clusters lasting **more than one month:**

1. **Intrusion Symptoms:** The trauma persistently intrudes into awareness.

    o Recurrent, involuntary, intrusive distressing memories.

    o Recurrent distressing dreams related to the trauma.

    o Dissociative reactions (flashbacks)[90] where the person feels/acts as if the trauma is recurring.

- Intense psychological distress at exposure to internal/external cues resembling an aspect of the trauma.

- Marked physiological reactions to those cues (e.g., heart pounding when hearing a car backfire if trauma involved an explosion).

2. **Persistent Avoidance:** Efforts to avoid distressing memories, thoughts, feelings, or external reminders associated with the trauma. This avoidance maintains the disorder.

3. **Negative Alterations in Cognitions and Mood:** Difficulty remembering important aspects of the trauma (dissociative amnesia), persistent negative beliefs about self/others/world ("I am bad," "No one can be trusted"), distorted blame of self or others, persistent negative emotional state (fear, horror, anger, guilt, shame), markedly diminished interest (anhedonia), feelings of detachment or estrangement from others, inability to experience positive emotions.

4. **Marked Alterations in Arousal and Reactivity:** Irritable behavior and angry outbursts, reckless or self-destructive behavior, hypervigilance (constantly[94] scanning for threats), exaggerated startle response, problems with concentration, sleep disturbance (difficulty falling/staying asleep, restless sleep).

These symptoms cause significant distress or impairment in functioning.

Acute Stress Disorder ASD

Acute Stress Disorder (ASD) shares the same trauma exposure criteria as PTSD. However, the symptom pattern (including intrusion, negative mood, dissociation, avoidance, arousal) occurs and resolves within the period of **3 days to 1 month** *following* **the traumatic event**. If the symptoms persist beyond one month and meet PTSD criteria, the diagnosis changes to PTSD. ASD can be seen as an immediate, acute reaction to trauma. Recognizing and intervening early with individuals experiencing ASD may help prevent the development of chronic PTSD.

Understanding Trauma Informed Care Principles

Trauma-Informed Care (TIC) is not a specific treatment model, but rather an organizational and clinical **approach** grounded in understanding the high prevalence of trauma and its potential impact on *everyone* seeking services. It operates on the assumption that anyone you encounter might have a history of trauma, visible or not, and adjusts practices accordingly to avoid re-traumatization and foster healing. It shifts the question from "What's wrong with you?" to **"What happened to you?"**

Core Principles of TIC (Text Description):

1. **Safety:** Creating environments where people feel physically and psychologically safe. This includes staff demeanor, predictability of routines, clear communication, and attention to physical setting.

2. **Trustworthiness and Transparency:** Building trust through clear expectations, consistent boundaries, explaining reasons for decisions, and being dependable. Operations and decisions are conducted with transparency to build and maintain trust.

3. **Peer Support:** Utilizing individuals with lived experience of trauma and recovery to offer support, hope, and collaboration.

4. **Collaboration and Mutuality:** Recognizing that healing happens in relationships and power is shared. Partnering

with individuals in their care planning, recognizing their strengths and experience. Leveling power differences between staff and clients.

5. **Empowerment, Voice, and Choice:** Helping individuals identify their strengths, build skills, and feel empowered in their recovery. Providing choices in treatment and honoring their voice. Staff recognize the importance of individuals having a sense of control.

6. **Cultural, Historical, and Gender Issues:** Actively moving past cultural stereotypes and biases. Offering access to gender-responsive services. Recognizing the impact of historical trauma (e.g., on specific cultural or racial groups) and tailoring services accordingly.

Implementing TIC means examining policies, procedures, staff training, and physical environments to ensure they align with these principles.

Brief Note on Dissociative Disorders

Dissociation is a disruption in the usually integrated functions of consciousness, memory, identity, or perception of the environment. It can be a defense mechanism during overwhelming trauma—a way of mentally "disconnecting" from a terrifying reality. While transient dissociative symptoms (like flashbacks or feeling detached) occur in PTSD/ASD, **Dissociative Disorders** involve more persistent or recurrent disruptions:[101]

- **Dissociative Identity Disorder (DID):** Formerly multiple personality disorder. Disruption of identity characterized by two or more distinct personality states ("alters"),[102] involving marked discontinuity in sense of self and agency, accompanied by alterations in affect, behavior, consciousness, memory, perception, cognition, and/or sensory-motor[103] functioning. Recurrent gaps in recall of everyday events, personal information,[105] or traumatic events.

- **Dissociative Amnesia:** Inability to recall important autobiographical information, usually of a traumatic or stressful nature, inconsistent with ordinary forgetting. May involve localized amnesia (loss of memory for specific period) or generalized amnesia (loss of identity/life history). May involve dissociative fugue (bewildered wandering or purposeful travel associated with amnesia).

- **Depersonalization/Derealization Disorder:** Persistent or recurrent experiences of depersonalization (feeling detached from[107] one's own thoughts, feelings, body; like an outside observer) and/or derealization (feeling the external world is unreal, dreamlike, foggy). Reality testing remains intact (person knows these feelings aren't objectively real).

Care for dissociative disorders is specialized, often involving long-term psychotherapy focused on integration and trauma processing. Nurses provide supportive care, safety, anxiety management, and reality orientation (for depersonalization/derealization).

Nursing Priorities Trauma and Dissociation

Whether dealing with diagnosed PTSD/ASD or simply applying a TIC approach universally, nursing priorities revolve around safety, trust, and empowerment.

1. **Safety and Security:**
   - **Assess Risk:** Screen for suicidal ideation, self-harm, risk-taking behaviors, potential for aggression (often linked to hyperarousal/startle).

o **Create Safe Environment:** Ensure physical safety. Provide psychological safety through predictability, clear communication, respecting personal space, avoiding sudden approaches. Be mindful of potential triggers in the environment (noise, certain smells, visual stimuli).

2. **Build Trusting Relationship:**

   o Be **patient, consistent, authentic, and respectful**. Trust may be difficult due to past betrayals associated with trauma.

   o **Explain** roles, procedures, and what to expect clearly. Avoid surprises.

   o **Offer choices** whenever possible to restore a sense of control.

3. **Manage Anxiety and Arousal:**

   o **Teach Grounding Techniques:** Help patients connect with the present moment during flashbacks or dissociation. Examples:

      ▪ *Sensory Grounding:* Focus on 5 things you see, 4 things you feel, 3 things you hear, 2 things you smell, 1 thing you taste. Holding ice, strong mints.

      ▪ *Mental Grounding:* Name categories (types of animals, colors), describe environment in detail.

   o **Relaxation Skills:** Deep breathing, progressive muscle relaxation.

   o **Manage Hypervigilance:** Acknowledge their need to feel safe; allow preferred seating (e.g., back to wall) if feasible and safe; explain unit safety measures.

4. **Address Avoidance (Carefully):**

   o Understand avoidance is a symptom, not defiance.

   o Gently encourage participation in therapeutic activities but don't force confrontation with trauma reminders before the patient is ready (this is usually done strategically in therapy).

5. **Promote Sleep:** Implement sleep hygiene measures; address nightmares (medication like Prazosin may be ordered).

6. **Encourage Expression (Patient-Paced):**

   o Allow patients to share their experiences *if and when they choose*. Listen non-judgmentally.

   o Focus on validating the *feelings* associated with the trauma.

   o Do not press for details of the trauma, as this can be re-traumatizing outside of a structured therapeutic context.

7. **Medication Education:** Explain purpose/side effects of prescribed medications (SSRIs/SNRIs common for PTSD; Prazosin for nightmares; anxiolytics used cautiously).

8. **Psychoeducation:** Teach about common trauma reactions, PTSD/ASD symptoms, the rationale for TIC, coping skills, treatment options (therapy like EMDR, CPT, Prolonged Exposure).

9. **Apply TIC Principles Consistently:** In every interaction, consider how to maximize safety, trust, collaboration, empowerment, and choice.

Trauma-Informed Care Principles Checklist (For Self-Reflection/Practice Guidance):

- Am I creating a sense of physical and psychological **Safety**? (Calm tone, predictable routine, respecting space?)

- Am I demonstrating **Trustworthiness & Transparency**? (Being consistent, explaining actions, being honest?)

- Am I facilitating **Peer Support** where possible? (Connecting to support groups or peer specialists?)

- Am I fostering **Collaboration & Mutuality**? (Asking for input, shared decision-making, acknowledging their expertise on themselves?)

- Am I promoting **Empowerment, Voice & Choice**? (Offering options, asking permission, highlighting strengths, respecting decisions?)

- Am I considering **Cultural, Historical & Gender Issues**? (Asking about cultural needs, being sensitive to potential historical trauma, using appropriate language?)

Case Snippet: PTSD

- *Scenario:* Ms. Jones, a combat veteran, is admitted for depression and reports intrusive memories of explosions, nightmares, avoidance of crowds, hypervigilance (always sits facing the door), and an exaggerated startle response to loud noises. She feels detached from her family and irritable.

- *Nursing Considerations:* Priorities include safety assessment (suicide risk), building trust slowly, applying

TIC principles consistently (approaching calmly, explaining actions, offering choices), teaching grounding techniques for flashbacks/intrusive memories, managing hyperarousal (allowing preferred seating if safe, teaching relaxation), psychoeducation about PTSD, medication management (e.g., SSRI, Prazosin), encouraging connection with veteran peer support groups, and collaborating with her therapist on treatment goals. Avoid asking for graphic details of combat unless she offers them within a therapeutic context.

Healing from Invisible Wounds

The impact of trauma can be profound and long-lasting, shaping an individual's worldview, relationships, and sense of self. Trauma-informed care provides a necessary framework for all healthcare interactions, recognizing that safety and trust are prerequisites for healing. For those with specific diagnoses like PTSD or ASD, nursing care focuses on managing distressing symptoms like intrusion and hyperarousal, fostering coping skills like grounding, supporting engagement in specialized therapies, and patiently rebuilding a sense of security and control. It's about acknowledging the reality of past hurts while empowering individuals to move forward. Finally, we'll look at conditions affecting cognition and the mind-body connection: neurocognitive and somatic disorders.

Core Learnings from This Section

- **Trauma/Stressor-Related Disorders (PTSD, ASD)** result from exposure to traumatic events.

- **PTSD:** Symptoms (intrusion, avoidance, negative alterations in cognition/mood, arousal/reactivity) persist >1 month.

- **ASD:** Similar symptoms occur within 3 days to 1 month post-trauma.

- **Trauma-Informed Care (TIC)** is an essential approach assuming potential trauma history; focuses on Safety, Trust, Collaboration, Empowerment, Choice, Cultural Sensitivity. Ask "What happened to you?"

- **Dissociative Disorders** involve disruptions in consciousness/memory/identity, often trauma-linked.

- **Nursing Priorities: Safety** (physical/psychological), building **Trust**, managing anxiety/arousal with **Grounding** techniques, **Trigger Awareness**, promoting **Sleep**, patient-paced **Expression**, applying **TIC** principles consistently.

Chapter 13 Neurocognitive and Somatic Disorders

Our final group of conditions involves two distinct areas: **Neurocognitive Disorders (NCDs)**, which affect the brain's ability to think, remember, and reason, and **Somatic Symptom and Related Disorders**, where psychological distress manifests primarily through physical symptoms. Both require careful assessment to differentiate from other conditions and specialized nursing approaches focused on safety, function, and managing the complex interplay between mind and body.

Delirium Versus Dementia Key Differences

Both delirium and dementia are NCDs involving a decline in cognitive function, but they are critically different in onset, course, and cause. Confusing them can lead to missed opportunities for treating a reversible condition (delirium).

Key Distinctions (Text Description):

- **Onset: Delirium** has an **acute or subacute onset**, developing over hours to days. **Dementia** has an **insidious onset**, developing gradually over months to years.

- **Course: Delirium** typically has a **fluctuating course** throughout the day, with symptoms often worsening in the evening ("sundowning"). **Dementia** usually involves a **slowly progressive decline** without dramatic daily fluctuations (though sundowning can also occur).

- **Duration: Delirium** is usually **temporary** (hours to weeks) and **reversible** if the underlying cause is treated. **Dementia** is typically **chronic, progressive, and irreversible** (though treatments can slow progression or manage symptoms).

- **Consciousness: Delirium** involves a **disturbance in consciousness** (reduced clarity of awareness of the environment). Patients may be drowsy, lethargic, or hyperalert and agitated. **Dementia** generally involves **clear consciousness** until the very late stages.

- **Attention: Impaired attention** (difficulty focusing, sustaining, or shifting attention) is a **hallmark feature of delirium** and often fluctuates. In **dementia**, attention is relatively **intact in the early stages** but becomes progressively impaired later.

- **Cause: Delirium** is always **caused by an underlying physiological disturbance**—a medical condition (infection, hypoxia, electrolyte imbalance, organ failure), substance intoxication or withdrawal, medication side effect, or toxin exposure. Finding and treating the cause is key. **Dementia** is caused by **primary brain pathology**, such as Alzheimer's disease, vascular disease, Lewy body disease, etc.

Why is distinguishing them so important? Delirium is often a medical emergency indicating a serious underlying problem that needs immediate identification and treatment. Assuming an acutely confused older patient just has worsening dementia could be fatal if they actually have delirium due to sepsis or hypoxia. **Always suspect delirium first in cases of acute cognitive change.**

Alzheimer's Disease Basics

Alzheimer's Disease (AD) is the most common cause of dementia, accounting for 60-80% of cases. It's a progressive neurodegenerative disease characterized by the buildup of amyloid plaques and neurofibrillary tangles in the brain, leading to nerve cell death and cognitive decline.

Key Features/Progression:

- **Early Stage (Mild):** Primarily memory loss, especially for recent events. Difficulty finding words, organizing/planning, misplacing things. Mood changes (irritability, anxiety) may occur. Functioning is often still relatively independent with some assistance.

- **Middle Stage (Moderate):** Memory loss worsens, affecting remote memory too. Increased confusion, disorientation to time/place. Language difficulties (aphasia) become more pronounced. Difficulty recognizing familiar people. Impaired judgment, impulse control. Changes in personality/behavior (agitation, wandering, suspiciousness, delusions) often emerge. Requires significant assistance with ADLs.

- **Late Stage (Severe):** Severe cognitive impairment. Loss of ability to communicate coherently, recognize loved ones, perform basic ADLs (feeding, toileting, bathing). Motor function declines (difficulty walking, swallowing). Requires total care. Increased susceptibility to infections (like pneumonia), which are often the cause of death.

While medications (cholinesterase inhibitors, memantine) can temporarily slow cognitive decline or manage symptoms for some, there is currently no cure for Alzheimer's disease.

Somatic Symptom and Related Disorders Overview

This group involves a primary focus on physical (somatic) symptoms associated with significant psychological distress and impairment. The key is that the distress and preoccupation are excessive or disproportionate to the physical symptoms themselves.

- **Somatic Symptom Disorder:** One or more distressing physical symptoms (like pain, fatigue, GI issues) that cause disruption in daily life, coupled with **excessive**

thoughts, feelings, or behaviors related to these symptoms. This might include:

- o Disproportionate/persistent thoughts about the seriousness of symptoms.

- o Persistently high levels of anxiety about health or symptoms.

- o Excessive time and energy devoted to symptoms or[130] health concerns (e.g., frequent doctor visits, researching). The focus is on the *psychological reaction* to the physical symptoms.

- **Conversion Disorder (Functional Neurological Symptom Disorder):** Symptoms involve altered voluntary motor or sensory function that suggest a neurological condition but are **incompatible** with recognized neurological or medical findings. Examples include weakness/paralysis, abnormal movements (tremors, gait disturbance), swallowing symptoms, speech symptoms (slurred speech, aphonia), seizures ("non-epileptic seizures"), numbness or sensory loss, special sensory symptoms (blindness, deafness). Symptoms are *not* intentionally produced or feigned. Often associated with preceding stress or psychological conflict.

Important Distinction: These are different from **Factitious Disorder** (intentionally feigning or inducing symptoms to assume the sick role) and **Malingering** (intentionally feigning symptoms for external gain, like disability benefits or avoiding work). In Somatic Symptom and Conversion disorders, the symptoms are experienced as real by the patient.

Nursing Priorities Neurocognitive Disorders Delirium Dementia

Priorities for Delirium:

1. **Identify and Treat Underlying Cause:** This is paramount and requires collaboration with the medical team. Monitor lab results, vital signs. Ensure prescribed treatments for the cause (e.g., antibiotics for infection) are administered.

2. **Safety:** High risk! Prevent falls, injuries, pulling out lines/tubes. Use lowest level of restraint necessary (environmental modifications, sitter preferred over physical restraints which can worsen agitation). Bed alarms, low bed position.

3. **Manage Confusion/Agitation:**

   o **Reorient frequently** and simply (person, place, time). Use clocks, calendars, familiar objects.

   o Maintain a **calm, quiet, well-lit** environment. Reduce excessive noise/stimulation.

   o Use **simple, direct communication**. Avoid complex explanations.

   o **Promote sleep-wake cycle:** Encourage daytime activity, minimize nighttime disturbances.

   o **Encourage Family Presence:** Familiar faces can be calming and help with orientation (if their presence is indeed calming).

4. **Physiological Stability:** Monitor hydration, nutrition, elimination. Assist as needed.

Priorities for Dementia (including Alzheimer's):

1. **Safety:** Prevent wandering (secure environment, ID bracelet), falls (remove hazards, appropriate footwear), accidental ingestion, burns. Ensure environment is safe and adapted to deficits.

2. **Promote Orientation (as able):** Use clocks, calendars, familiar objects, labels. Maintain routines. Avoid constant quizzing ("Do you know who I am?") if it causes distress.

3. **Communication Strategies:**

   o Use a **calm, positive tone**. Approach from the front.

   o Use **simple sentences, concrete words**. Speak slowly.

   o Allow **ample time** for processing and response.

   o Use **nonverbal cues** (gestures, touch - if appropriate).

   o **Avoid arguing** or confronting disorientation/false beliefs, especially in later stages. Use **validation** and **redirection**.

4. **Validation Therapy:** Focus on the *feeling* or *need* behind the patient's words or behavior, rather than correcting the factual inaccuracy. If a patient asks for their long-deceased mother, instead of saying "Your mother died years ago," try "You miss your mother. Tell me about her." This acknowledges the emotion and reduces distress.

5. **Manage Behavioral Symptoms (Agitation, Aggression, Wandering):**

   o Look for **underlying causes/triggers** (pain, hunger, thirst, need to toilet, constipation, infection, fear, overstimulation, boredom). Address the unmet need.

   o Use **redirection** to a different activity or topic.

- Maintain a **calm, structured routine**.

- Use **music therapy, reminiscence therapy, simple activities**.

- Use medications for behavior cautiously and only when non-pharmacological approaches fail.

6. **Promote Dignity and Function:**

- Encourage **independence** in ADLs as much as possible. Break tasks into small steps. Provide cues.

- Maintain **personhood**. Address patient by name, interact respectfully, involve them in simple decisions.

- Support **continence** (scheduled toileting).

- Ensure adequate **nutrition/hydration** (finger foods, adaptive utensils, supplements if needed).

7. **Family/Caregiver Support:** Provide education about the disease, behavioral management strategies, community resources (support groups, respite care, legal/financial planning). Acknowledge caregiver burden.

Nursing Priorities Somatic Symptom and Conversion Disorders

1. **Rule Out/Manage Medical Conditions:** Ensure a thorough medical workup has been done. Address any co-existing medical issues.

2. **Build Therapeutic Relationship:** Acknowledge the symptom is real *to the patient*. Avoid implying "it's all in your head." Build trust through empathy and consistent care.

3. **Limit Reinforcement of Sick Role:** Provide necessary care for physical symptoms but minimize excessive

attention or special privileges related to the symptoms. Encourage functional behavior.

4. **Shift Focus to Feelings and Coping:** Gradually shift conversation away from detailed somatic complaints towards exploring feelings, life stressors, and coping mechanisms. Ask: "How has this symptom affected your life?" "What was going on around the time this symptom started?"

5. **Stress Management/Relaxation:** Teach techniques like deep breathing, mindfulness, progressive muscle relaxation to help manage underlying anxiety or stress.

6. **Assertiveness Training:** Help patients learn to express needs and feelings directly rather than through physical symptoms.

7. **Promote Independence in ADLs:** Encourage self-care and participation in activities despite physical symptoms (within safe limits). Set realistic goals for increasing activity.

8. **Collaborate with Team:** Work closely with physicians, therapists (CBT is often helpful), physical therapists (for conversion symptoms) to ensure a consistent approach.

9. **Maintain Realistic Expectations:** Improvement may be gradual. Focus on improved functioning and coping rather than complete symptom elimination.

Case Snippet: Conversion Disorder

- *Scenario:* Mrs. Chen, 40, presents to the ED with sudden paralysis of her left leg after a major argument with her husband about finances. Extensive neurological workup (MRI, nerve conduction studies) is completely normal. She expresses distress about the paralysis but seems relatively unconcerned about the underlying cause (la belle indifférence - though not always present).

- *Nursing Considerations:* After medical causes are ruled out, priorities include acknowledging the reality of her experience ("It must be frightening not being able to move your leg"), ensuring safety (fall precautions), encouraging self-care within limitations, focusing care away from the paralyzed limb (avoiding excessive attention/massage), gently exploring stressors around the time of onset without directly linking it to the paralysis initially, teaching basic anxiety reduction techniques, and collaborating with therapy/PT for functional rehabilitation. Avoid suggesting she isn't trying or that it's "fake."

Mind, Brain, and Body Interconnected

This final group of disorders underscores the profound connections between our brain's cognitive functions, our psychological state, and our physical bodies. Delirium reminds us that acute changes in thinking often signal underlying medical emergencies. Dementia highlights the devastating impact of progressive brain disease, requiring care focused on safety, dignity, and function. Somatic symptom and conversion disorders reveal how psychological distress can manifest physically, demanding care that acknowledges the physical complaint while addressing the underlying emotional turmoil and coping mechanisms. Across all these conditions, nursing requires careful assessment, a focus on safety, collaboration with the medical team, and compassionate support for both patients and their families navigating these complex challenges.

Core Learnings from This Section

- **Neurocognitive Disorders (NCDs)** affect cognitive function (thinking, memory).

- **Delirium:** Acute onset, fluctuating course, altered consciousness/attention, *caused by underlying medical issue* (reversible if cause treated). Priority: Identify/treat cause, ensure safety.

- **Dementia (e.g., Alzheimer's):** Gradual onset, progressive course, clear consciousness (early), *caused by primary brain pathology* (irreversible). Priority: Safety, function, dignity, communication (Validation), family support.

- **Distinguish Delirium from Dementia:** Acute change = Suspect Delirium first!

- **Somatic Symptom & Related Disorders:** Physical symptoms linked to excessive psychological distress/preoccupation (Somatic Symptom Disorder) or neurological symptoms incompatible with medical findings (Conversion Disorder). Symptoms are *not* intentionally produced.

- **Nursing Priorities (Somatic/Conversion):** Rule out medical causes, build trust, acknowledge symptom reality (to patient), shift focus to feelings/coping, limit sick role reinforcement, promote function.

Part 3: Treatment Modalities & The Nursing Process

Chapter 14 Psychopharmacology Essentials for Nurses

Medications are powerful tools in managing mental health conditions. They can significantly reduce distressing symptoms, improve functioning, and facilitate engagement in other therapies. However, they are not magic bullets, and their use requires careful consideration, monitoring, and education. As a nurse, your role goes far beyond simply administering pills. You are on the front lines of assessing effectiveness, identifying side effects—some merely inconvenient, others potentially life-threatening—and educating patients and families to ensure safe and effective use. This section provides a simplified overview of the major drug classes, focusing on what you *need to know* for clinical practice.

Major Drug Classes Simplified

We group psychiatric medications based on their primary intended use or mechanism, though there's often overlap in what they treat.

1. Antidepressants:

- **Primary Use:** Treating Major Depressive Disorder, Persistent Depressive Disorder, Anxiety Disorders (GAD, Panic, Social Anxiety, OCD), PTSD.

- **Key Classes & Examples (Simplified Info):**

    - **Selective Serotonin Reuptake Inhibitors (SSRIs):** (e.g., fluoxetine, sertraline, citalopram, escitalopram). *How they work (simply):* Increase serotonin levels by blocking its "reuptake" or reabsorption, making more available in the synapse. *Need-to-know:* Generally first-line due to better side effect profile and safety in overdose compared to older agents. Common side effects include GI upset (nausea, diarrhea -

189

often temporary), headache, insomnia or sedation, and **sexual dysfunction** (decreased libido, difficulty achieving orgasm - often persistent and a major reason for non-adherence). Risk of **Serotonin Syndrome**.

- o **Serotonin-Norepinephrine Reuptake Inhibitors (SNRIs):** (e.g., venlafaxine, duloxetine, desvenlafaxine). *How they work (simply):* Increase both serotonin and norepinephrine levels by blocking their reuptake. *Need-to-know:* Similar side effects to SSRIs, but may also cause increased blood pressure or pulse (due to norepinephrine). Can be helpful for neuropathic pain as well (duloxetine). Risk of **Serotonin Syndrome**. Venlafaxine, especially, can cause significant withdrawal symptoms if stopped abruptly.

- o **Tricyclic Antidepressants (TCAs):** (e.g., amitriptyline, nortriptyline, imipramine). *How they work (simply):* Older class, block reuptake of norepinephrine and serotonin, but also block other receptors (muscarinic, histamine, alpha-adrenergic). *Need-to-know:* Effective, but have more side effects due to less specific action: **anticholinergic effects** (dry mouth, constipation, blurred vision, urinary retention), **orthostatic hypotension** (dizziness upon standing - fall risk!), sedation, weight gain, **cardiac effects** (arrhythmias - obtain baseline EKG). **Highly lethal in overdose** - use with caution in suicidal patients.

- o **Monoamine Oxidase Inhibitors (MAOIs):** (e.g., phenelzine, tranylcypromine, selegiline patch).*How they work (simply):* Older class,

190

inhibit the enzyme (MAO) that breaks down serotonin, norepinephrine, and dopamine, increasing their levels. *Need-to-know:* Very effective but less used due to significant safety concerns. Require strict adherence to a **tyramine-restricted diet** (avoid aged cheeses, cured meats, fermented foods, etc.) to prevent **Hypertensive Crisis**. Numerous potentially fatal **drug interactions** (e.g., with most other antidepressants, certain pain meds like meperidine, decongestants). Usually reserved for treatment-resistant depression.

- o **Atypical Antidepressants:** Miscellaneous group with unique mechanisms.

    - *Bupropion:* Blocks reuptake of norepinephrine and dopamine. Activating (can cause insomnia, anxiety), less likely to cause sexual dysfunction or weight gain. Also used for smoking cessation. Lowers seizure threshold - contraindicated in seizure disorders or eating disorders (due to electrolyte imbalance risk).

    - *Mirtazapine:* Enhances serotonin/norepinephrine release, also blocks histamine receptors. Often causes significant sedation (taken at bedtime) and weight gain/increased appetite. Fewer sexual side effects.

    - *Trazodone:* Primarily blocks serotonin receptors and histamine receptors. Mainly used at lower doses as a **sleep aid** due to potent sedation. Risk of **priapism** (prolonged, painful erection - medical emergency!).

2. Antipsychotics:

- **Primary Use:** Treating psychosis (symptoms like hallucinations, delusions, disorganized thinking) in Schizophrenia, Schizoaffective Disorder, Bipolar Mania. Also used as mood stabilizers, for agitation, and sometimes adjunctively in depression.

- **Key Classes & Examples:**

    o **Typical (First-Generation/Conventional) Antipsychotics (FGAs):** (e.g., haloperidol, chlorpromazine). *How they work (simply):* Primarily block dopamine D2 receptors strongly. *Need-to-know:* Very effective for positive symptoms of psychosis. High risk of **Extrapyramidal Symptoms (EPS)** including acute dystonia, akathisia, parkinsonism. Higher risk of **Tardive Dyskinesia (TD)** with long-term use. Also risk of **Neuroleptic Malignant Syndrome (NMS)**. Sedation and anticholinergic effects vary by agent (chlorpromazine more sedating/anticholinergic, haloperidol less so but higher EPS risk).

    o **Atypical (Second-Generation) Antipsychotics (SGAs):** (e.g., risperidone, olanzapine, quetiapine, ziprasidone, aripiprazole, lurasidone, clozapine). *How they work (simply):* Block dopamine D2 receptors (often less intensely than FGAs) and also block serotonin 2A receptors. *Need-to-know:* Generally effective for positive symptoms, may have some benefit for negative symptoms. Lower risk of EPS and TD compared to FGAs (but risk is still present, especially at

192

higher doses). **Higher risk of Metabolic Syndrome** (significant weight gain, increased blood glucose/risk of diabetes, dyslipidemia). Requires regular monitoring. Other side effects vary: sedation (olanzapine, quetiapine), orthostatic hypotension, hyperprolactinemia (risperidone). **Clozapine** is uniquely effective for treatment-resistant schizophrenia but carries risk of **agranulocytosis** (severe low white blood cell count), requiring strict blood monitoring (REMS program). Risk of **NMS** exists with all antipsychotics.

3. Mood Stabilizers:

- **Primary Use:** Treating Bipolar Disorder (managing acute mania/depression, preventing future episodes). Sometimes used for impulse control disorders, aggression.

- **Key Agents & Examples:**

  - **Lithium:** *How it works (simply):* Mechanism complex and not fully understood, affects neurotransmitter systems and intracellular signaling. *Need-to-know:* Very effective, especially for classic euphoric mania and suicide prevention in bipolar disorder. **Narrow therapeutic range** (typically 0.6-1.2 mEq/L) - requires regular blood level monitoring. **Toxicity** is a major concern (mild: tremor, nausea, thirst; moderate: confusion, ataxia, slurred speech; severe: seizures, coma, death). Requires adequate hydration and consistent salt intake. Long-term risks include thyroid dysfunction (hypothyroidism) and kidney problems. Common side effects: tremor, increased thirst/urination, weight gain, GI upset.

- o **Anticonvulsants:** Several drugs originally developed for epilepsy are effective mood stabilizers.

  - *Valproic Acid (Depakote): How it works (simply):* Increases GABA effects, affects sodium channels. *Need-to-know:* Effective for acute mania, mixed states, maintenance. Requires monitoring of blood levels, liver function tests (LFTs), complete blood count (CBC - risk of thrombocytopenia). Common SEs: GI upset, sedation, weight gain, tremor, hair loss. **Hepatotoxicity** and **pancreatitis** are rare but serious risks. Highly teratogenic (avoid in pregnancy).

  - *Carbamazepine (Tegretol): How it works (simply):* Affects sodium channels. *Need-to-know:* Effective for mania, mixed states. Induces its own metabolism (requires dose adjustments). Can cause bone marrow suppression (monitor CBC - risk of agranulocytosis/aplastic anemia, though rare). Many drug interactions. Common SEs: dizziness, drowsiness, GI upset. Risk of Stevens-Johnson Syndrome (SJS).

  - *Lamotrigine (Lamictal): How it works (simply):* Affects sodium channels, may modulate glutamate. *Need-to-know:* Particularly effective for preventing bipolar *depression*. Not very effective for

194

acute mania. Main concern is **Stevens-Johnson Syndrome (SJS)**, a potentially life-threatening rash. Requires **slow dose titration** to minimize SJS risk. Educate patients to report any rash immediately.

4. Anxiolytics (Anti-Anxiety Medications):

- **Primary Use:** Treating anxiety symptoms, anxiety disorders, insomnia, acute agitation, alcohol withdrawal.

- **Key Classes & Examples:**

  - **Benzodiazepines (BZDs):** (e.g., diazepam, lorazepam, alprazolam, clonazepam). *How they work (simply):* Enhance the effects of GABA, the brain's main inhibitory neurotransmitter, causing sedation and relaxation. *Need-to-know:* Work quickly, effective for short-term relief of severe anxiety or panic. High potential for **tolerance, dependence, and addiction. Withdrawal syndrome** can be severe and potentially life-threatening (seizures, delirium), requiring slow tapering. Cause sedation, dizziness, impaired coordination/cognition (risk of falls, accidents). Effects potentiated by alcohol/other CNS depressants (risk of respiratory depression/overdose). Ideally used short-term or PRN, not for chronic anxiety management.

  - **Buspirone:** *How it works (simply):* Non-BZD, affects serotonin receptors. *Need-to-know:* Takes weeks to become effective (like antidepressants). Does not cause sedation, dependence, or withdrawal. Not effective PRN. Used for GAD. Generally well-tolerated (dizziness, headache, nausea possible).

- Other Agents: Antidepressants (SSRIs/SNRIs) are first-line for long-term treatment of most anxiety disorders. **Beta-blockers** (e.g., propranolol) can help with physical symptoms of performance anxiety (stage fright). **Antihistamines** (e.g., hydroxyzine) used for sedative/anxiolytic effects, non-addictive.

5. Stimulants:

- **Primary Use:** Treating Attention-Deficit/Hyperactivity Disorder (ADHD). Also used for narcolepsy.

- **Key Agents & Examples:** (Methylphenidate - Ritalin, Concerta; Amphetamine salts - Adderall; Lisdexamfetamine - Vyvanse). *How they work (simply):* Increase levels of dopamine and norepinephrine in areas of the brain involved in attention and impulse control. *Need-to-know:* Effective in improving focus and reducing hyperactivity/impulsivity. Common side effects include **insomnia** (give earlier in day), **appetite suppression** (monitor weight/growth in children), headache, irritability, potential increase in BP/pulse. High potential for **misuse, abuse, and diversion**. Schedule II controlled substances.

Need to Know Mechanisms of Action Simplified

You don't need to be a neuroscientist, but understanding the basics helps. Most psychotropic drugs work by altering **neurotransmission**—how nerve cells (neurons) communicate using chemical messengers called **neurotransmitters**. Key players include:

- **Serotonin:** Involved in mood, anxiety, sleep, appetite, obsession/compulsion. Low levels linked to depression/anxiety. SSRIs/SNRIs increase serotonin.

- **Norepinephrine:** Involved in alertness, energy, attention, mood, stress response. Low levels linked to depression/fatigue; excess linked to anxiety/mania. SNRIs/TCAs/Bupropion affect norepinephrine.

- **Dopamine:** Involved in motivation, pleasure/reward, movement, attention, psychosis. Low levels linked to Parkinson's, possibly negative symptoms/depression; excess linked to psychosis/mania. Antipsychotics primarily block dopamine; stimulants increase it.

- **GABA (Gamma-aminobutyric acid):** The main *inhibitory* neurotransmitter—it calms nerve activity. Benzodiazepines enhance GABA's effects, causing relaxation/sedation.

Drugs can work by:

- **Blocking Reuptake:** Preventing the neurotransmitter from being reabsorbed by the sending neuron, leaving more in the synapse (gap between neurons) to act on the receiving neuron (e.g., SSRIs, SNRIs).

- **Blocking Receptors:** Preventing the neurotransmitter from binding to the receiving neuron's receptor, thus blocking its effect (e.g., antipsychotics blocking dopamine receptors).

- **Inhibiting Enzymes:** Preventing the breakdown of the neurotransmitter (e.g., MAOIs inhibiting MAO enzyme).

- **Enhancing Neurotransmitter Action:** Making the neurotransmitter work more effectively (e.g., benzodiazepines enhancing GABA).

Common and Serious Side Effects Focus on Recognition and Action

Safe nursing care hinges on recognizing side effects and knowing when to act. Some are common annoyances; others are emergencies.

Common (Often Manageable) Side Effects & Basic Management:

- **GI Upset (Nausea, Diarrhea):** Common with SSRIs/SNRIs initially. *Action:* Take with food, usually improves over time.

- **Headache:** Common with SSRIs/SNRIs. *Action:* Simple analgesics, usually improves.

- **Sedation:** Common with TCAs, mirtazapine, trazodone, some antipsychotics/anxiolytics. *Action:* Take at bedtime, caution driving/operating machinery.

- **Insomnia:** Common with SSRIs, SNRIs, bupropion, stimulants. *Action:* Take dose earlier in day, practice sleep hygiene, short-term sleep aid if needed.

- **Dry Mouth (Anticholinergic):** Common with TCAs, some antipsychotics. *Action:* Sugar-free candy/gum, frequent sips of water, good oral hygiene.

- **Constipation (Anticholinergic):** Common with TCAs, some antipsychotics. *Action:* Increase fluids/fiber, exercise, stool softeners if needed.

- **Blurred Vision (Anticholinergic):** Usually temporary. *Action:* Caution driving, may need reading glasses temporarily. If sudden/severe, could indicate glaucoma (rare).

- **Orthostatic Hypotension:** Common with TCAs, some antipsychotics (esp. clozapine, risperidone). *Action:* Rise slowly from sitting/lying, stay hydrated, monitor BP, fall precautions.

- **Weight Gain:** Common with mirtazapine, olanzapine, TCAs, lithium, valproic acid. *Action:* Monitor weight, educate on diet/exercise.

- **Sexual Dysfunction:** Common with SSRIs/SNRIs. *Action:* Encourage reporting (patients often embarrassed), discuss potential strategies with prescriber (dose reduction, drug holidays, switching meds, adding bupropion).

Serious Side Effects ("Red Flag" Boxes - Text Description):

- **RED FLAG: Neuroleptic Malignant Syndrome (NMS)**

  o *What it is:* Rare but potentially fatal reaction to antipsychotics (more common with FGAs but can occur with SGAs).

  o *Key Signs:* **F**ever (often very high), **E**ncephalopathy (confusion, altered consciousness), **V**ital sign instability (tachycardia, labile BP, tachypnea), **E**levated enzymes (CPK markedly high), **R**igidity ("lead pipe" muscle rigidity).

  o *Nurse Action:* **MEDICAL EMERGENCY!** Hold antipsychotic, notify provider STAT, transfer to medical unit likely needed, initiate supportive care (cooling blankets, IV fluids, vital sign monitoring), monitor labs (CPK, WBC). Dantrolene or bromocriptine may be ordered.

- **RED FLAG: Serotonin Syndrome**

  o *What it is:* Potentially life-threatening condition caused by excess serotonergic activity, usually involving multiple drugs (e.g., SSRI + MAOI, SSRI + St. John's Wort, SSRI + certain pain meds).

- *Key Signs (Triad):* **Mental status changes** (agitation, confusion, restlessness, lethargy, coma), **Autonomic hyperactivity** (fever, tachycardia, diaphoresis, diarrhea, shivering, hypertension), **Neuromuscular abnormalities** (tremor, hyperreflexia, myoclonus - muscle jerks, rigidity). Use mnemonic **SHIVERS**: Shivering, Hyperreflexia, Increased temperature, Vital sign instability, Encephalopathy, Restlessness, Sweating.

- *Nurse Action:* Hold suspected agent(s), notify provider STAT, provide supportive care (cooling, hydration, monitor vital signs), benzodiazepines for agitation/myoclonus. Usually resolves quickly once offending drugs stopped. Education on drug interactions is key.

- **RED FLAG: Hypertensive Crisis (with MAOIs)**
  - *What it is:* Dangerous spike in blood pressure due to interaction between MAOI and tyramine-containing foods or contraindicated medications.

  - *Key Signs:* Severe occipital headache, extremely high BP, palpitations, stiff neck, sweating, nausea/vomiting. Can lead to stroke.

  - *Nurse Action:* **MEDICAL EMERGENCY!** Hold MAOI, notify provider STAT, monitor BP closely, administer rapid-acting antihypertensive (e.g., phentolamine, nifedipine) as ordered. Prevention via strict diet/medication adherence is crucial.

- **RED FLAG: Extrapyramidal Symptoms (EPS) & Tardive Dyskinesia (TD)**

- *EPS:* Acute Dystonia (sudden muscle spasms - neck, eyes, back; frightening!), Akathisia (intense inner restlessness, inability to sit still), Parkinsonism (tremor, rigidity, slow movement). *Nurse Action:* Assess using scales (like Abnormal Involuntary Movement Scale - AIMS, periodically for TD risk), notify provider. Administer anticholinergics (benztropine, diphenhydramine) or beta-blockers (for akathisia) as ordered for acute EPS.

- *TD:* Involuntary movements, often face/tongue/lips (lip smacking, grimacing, choreoathetoid movements of limbs/trunk). Often appears after long-term use, can be irreversible. *Nurse Action:* Regular AIMS screening is essential for early detection. Notify provider immediately if TD suspected (may need dose reduction or switch). Prevention involves using lowest effective antipsychotic dose and preferring SGAs where possible.

- **RED FLAG: Agranulocytosis (with Clozapine)**

  - *What it is:* Potentially fatal drop in white blood cells (neutrophils), increasing infection risk.

  - *Key Signs:* Flu-like symptoms (fever, sore throat, malaise). May have no symptoms initially.

  - *Nurse Action:* Strict adherence to WBC monitoring protocol (ANC checks weekly initially, then biweekly, then monthly). Educate patient intensely to report *any* sign of infection immediately for stat bloodwork. Hold clozapine and notify provider if ANC drops below threshold.

- **RED FLAG: Lithium Toxicity**

  - *What it is:* Lithium levels above therapeutic range (narrow window!). Can be caused by dehydration, decreased GFR, NSAID use, thiazide diuretics, low salt intake.

  - *Key Signs:* Mild (early): Fine tremor worsens, nausea, polyuria, thirst. Moderate: Coarse tremor, confusion, slurred speech, ataxia, lethargy, vomiting/diarrhea. Severe: Seizures, coma, cardiovascular collapse, death.

  - *Nurse Action:* Hold lithium, notify provider STAT, obtain stat lithium level, push fluids (if appropriate), monitor vital signs/neurological status closely. Hemodialysis may be needed for severe toxicity. Emphasize consistent fluid/salt intake to patients.

- **RED FLAG: Stevens-Johnson Syndrome (SJS) / Toxic Epidermal Necrolysis (TEN)**

  - *What it is:* Rare but severe, potentially fatal skin reaction, often associated with lamotrigine (especially with rapid dose increase) and carbamazepine.

  - *Key Signs:* Begins with flu-like symptoms followed by painful rash, blistering, skin detachment.

  - *Nurse Action:* **MEDICAL EMERGENCY!** Hold suspected drug, notify provider immediately. Requires hospitalization, often in burn unit. Educate patients (esp. on lamotrigine/carbamazepine) to report **any rash** immediately.

Patient Education Priorities

Effective patient education is arguably one of the most important nursing interventions in psychopharmacology. It promotes adherence, enhances safety, and empowers patients. Key areas include:

1. **Medication Name, Dose, Purpose:** Why are they taking it? What is it supposed to do?

2. **Timing and Administration:** When and how to take it (with food? bedtime?).

3. **Therapeutic Lag Time:** Especially for antidepressants/mood stabilizers – manage expectations, encourage patience.

4. **Importance of Adherence:** Taking it consistently as prescribed.

5. **NOT Stopping Abruptly:** Warn about discontinuation syndromes (SSRIs/SNRIs, venlafaxine especially) or withdrawal (BZDs).

6. **Common Side Effects:** What to expect, how to manage them (often temporary).

7. **Serious Side Effects:** What specific signs/symptoms require immediate reporting ("Red Flags"). Provide written info.

8. **Specific Precautions:** Dietary restrictions (MAOIs), need for bloodwork (lithium, clozapine, anticonvulsants), avoiding alcohol/other CNS depressants, effects on driving/machinery.

9. **Drug Interactions:** Importance of informing all providers (including dentists) about all medications, including OTC and herbal supplements (e.g., St. John's Wort).

10. **Role in Overall Treatment:** Medication helps manage symptoms but works best combined with therapy, coping skills, lifestyle changes. It's usually not a "cure."

11. **Questions/Contact:** Who to call if questions or problems arise.

Use clear, simple language. Avoid jargon. Use teach-back ("Can you tell me in your own words how you're going to take this medication?"). Provide written materials. Involve family members if appropriate and patient consents.

Final Thoughts on Pharmacology

Psychotropic medications have revolutionized mental health care, offering relief to many who previously had few options. But they are complex agents with significant potential for both benefit and harm. The nurse stands as a critical checkpoint—administering medications safely, diligently monitoring for therapeutic effects and adverse reactions (especially the dangerous ones!), and empowering patients with the knowledge they need to be active partners in their treatment. It requires continuous learning and vigilance, but skilled nursing care is indispensable for optimizing the outcomes of psychopharmacological treatment. Now that we've covered medications, let's look at other important treatment approaches.

Core Learnings from This Section

- Nurses play a key role in **assessment, monitoring, and education** related to psychotropic medications.

- Major classes include **Antidepressants** (SSRIs, SNRIs, TCAs, MAOIs, Atypicals), **Antipsychotics** (Typicals/FGAs,

Atypicals/SGAs), **Mood Stabilizers** (Lithium, Anticonvulsants), **Anxiolytics** (Benzodiazepines, Buspirone), and **Stimulants**.

- Understand simplified mechanisms (neurotransmitters like Serotonin, Dopamine, Norepinephrine, GABA) and basic drug actions (reuptake block, receptor block, etc.).

- **Prioritize recognition and action for serious side effects:** NMS, Serotonin Syndrome, Hypertensive Crisis, EPS/TD, Agranulocytosis, Lithium Toxicity, SJS. Know the key signs and immediate nursing actions.

- **Patient education is crucial** for adherence and safety: cover purpose, dose, timing, lag time, adherence, side effects (common vs. serious), precautions, interactions, role in treatment.

•

Chapter 15:Overview of Therapeutic Modalities

While medication often forms the bedrock of treatment for many mental health conditions, it's rarely the whole story. Recovery and improved quality of life usually depend on learning new ways of thinking, feeling, behaving, and relating to others. This is where psychosocial treatments—therapeutic modalities beyond medication—come in. These range from structured psychotherapies to group work to brain stimulation techniques. As a nurse, you won't typically conduct formal psychotherapy (unless you have advanced training), but understanding these modalities helps you support patients, reinforce skills, and contribute effectively to the interprofessional treatment plan.

Brief Introduction to Psychotherapy

Psychotherapy, or "talk therapy," involves regularly meeting with a trained therapist (psychologist, psychiatrist, licensed clinical social worker, psychiatric nurse practitioner, etc.) to explore thoughts, feelings, behaviors, and relationships to alleviate distress and improve functioning. There are many different types, often tailored to specific problems. Here are two highly influential approaches you'll often hear about:

Cognitive Behavioral Therapy (CBT):

- **Core Concept:** Our **thoughts** (cognitions) significantly influence our **feelings** and **behaviors**. Psychological distress often arises from distorted or unhelpful thinking patterns and learned maladaptive behaviors.

- **Focus:** Identifying negative or inaccurate thought patterns (e.g., overgeneralization, catastrophizing, black-and-white thinking), challenging these thoughts (cognitive restructuring), and replacing them with more realistic and adaptive ones. Also focuses on changing problematic behaviors through techniques like behavioral activation (scheduling positive activities for depression), exposure (for anxiety/phobias), and skills training.

- **Style:** Structured, goal-oriented, collaborative, often involves homework assignments. Focuses more on current problems than deep past exploration (though past influences are acknowledged).

- **Uses:** Highly effective for depression, anxiety disorders, OCD, eating disorders, insomnia, and more.

- **Nurse's Role:** While not conducting CBT, nurses can:

    o **Reinforce CBT skills:** Encourage patients to use thought records, challenge negative self-talk identified in therapy, or practice exposure homework.

    o **Identify Negative Thinking:** Notice and gently point out cognitive distortions in patient conversations ("It sounds like you're assuming the worst will happen. What's another possibility?").

    o **Promote Behavioral Activation:** Encourage depressed patients to engage in scheduled activities, even small ones.

    o **Support Exposure:** Provide encouragement and anxiety management support for patients facing feared situations as part of their therapy plan.

Dialectical Behavior Therapy (DBT):

- **Core Concept:** Finding a balance (the "dialectic") between **acceptance** (accepting oneself, reality, and emotions) and **change** (learning skills to change behaviors and manage emotions effectively). Originally developed for Borderline Personality Disorder (BPD), especially individuals with self-harm and suicidality.

- **Focus:** Teaching specific skills in four modules:

  1. **Mindfulness:** Paying attention non-judgmentally to the present moment (thoughts, feelings, sensations, environment). Helps increase self-awareness and decrease reactivity.

  2. **Distress Tolerance:** Learning to survive crises and accept reality without making things worse (e.g., using self-soothing, distraction, radical acceptance).

  3. **Emotion Regulation:** Understanding emotions, reducing emotional vulnerability, changing unwanted emotions.

  4. **Interpersonal Effectiveness:** Learning to assert needs effectively, maintain relationships, and preserve self-respect in interactions (using skills like DEAR MAN, GIVE, FAST).

- **Style:** Involves both individual therapy and group skills training. Emphasizes validation and a non-judgmental stance from the therapist.

- **Uses:** Standard treatment for BPD. Also adapted for substance use, eating disorders, PTSD, treatment-resistant depression.

- **Nurse's Role:**

  o **Understand DBT Principles:** Know the skills modules, understand the concept of dialectics and validation.

  o **Reinforce Skills:** Encourage patients to use specific DBT skills (e.g., "This seems like a good time to use a distress tolerance skill. Which one feels right?"). Coach them through using skills during moments of distress on the unit.

- ○ **Validate Effectively:** Practice validating patients' emotions and experiences ("It makes sense you would feel angry given what happened") without necessarily agreeing with maladaptive behaviors.

- ○ **Manage Crisis Behavior Consistent with DBT:** Focus on skills coaching rather than solely reactive limit-setting when possible. Collaborate with DBT therapist.

Group Therapy Basics

Group therapy brings together several individuals (usually 6-12) with similar issues or goals, guided by one or more therapists. It harnesses the power of group dynamics to facilitate change and support.

Types of Groups:

- **Psychoeducational Groups:** Focus on providing information about disorders, treatments, medications, coping skills (e.g., stress management group, medication education group, relapse prevention group). Often led by nurses on inpatient units.

- **Skills Training Groups:** Focus on teaching specific skills (e.g., DBT skills group, social skills training group, assertiveness training group). Structured with clear objectives.

- **Support Groups:** Members share experiences, provide mutual support, and reduce feelings of isolation around a common problem (e.g., grief support group, substance abuse recovery group like AA/NA - though often peer-led rather than therapist-led).

- **Interpersonal Process Groups:** Less structured, focus on exploring interpersonal dynamics *within the group* as they happen. Members learn about their own patterns of relating by interacting with others in the here-and-now. Requires specialized therapist training.

Therapeutic Factors in Groups (Yalom's Factors): Groups offer unique benefits:

- **Instillation of Hope:** Seeing others improve is inspiring.

- **Universality:** Realizing "I'm not alone" reduces shame and isolation.

- **Imparting Information:** Learning from therapist and peers.

- **Altruism:** Gaining self-esteem by helping others in the group.

- **Corrective Recapitulation of the Primary Family Group:** Re-experiencing and potentially resolving early family conflicts within the group structure.

- **Development of Socializing Techniques:** Practicing communication and relationship skills in a safe environment.

- **Imitative Behavior:** Learning by observing therapist and peers.

- **Interpersonal Learning:** Gaining insight into one's own interpersonal style and impact on others.

- **Group Cohesiveness:** Feeling of belonging, acceptance, and validation within the group (a powerful agent of change).

- **Catharsis:** Releasing strong emotions in a supportive environment.

210

- **Existential Factors:** Confronting universal life issues like death, freedom, responsibility, meaning.

Nurse's Role in Groups:

- **Lead/Co-lead Groups:** Especially psychoeducational and skills groups, depending on training and setting. Requires group leadership skills (facilitation, managing dynamics, time management).

- **Encourage Attendance:** Explain benefits, address patient reluctance.

- **Prepare Patients:** Briefly explain group purpose and expectations.

- **Process After Group:** Talk with patients individually about their experience in group, what they learned, any difficulties.

- **Maintain Confidentiality:** Reinforce group rules about confidentiality (what's said in group stays in group).

- **Manage Milieu:** Ensure unit environment supports group therapy (e.g., minimizing interruptions). Collaborate with group therapists.

Other Therapies Brain Stimulation Techniques

Sometimes, talk therapy and medication aren't enough, especially for severe or treatment-resistant conditions. Brain stimulation therapies directly affect brain activity.

Electroconvulsive Therapy (ECT):

- **What it is:** Medically induced brief seizure under general anesthesia and muscle relaxation. Typically given 2-3 times per week for a course of 6-12 treatments (sometimes more, sometimes maintenance).

- **Uses:** Highly effective for **severe major depression** (especially with psychotic features, catatonia, or acute suicidality), **mania**, and sometimes catatonia related to schizophrenia. Often used when rapid response is needed or medications have failed/are poorly tolerated.

- **Mechanism:** Not fully understood, but thought to cause changes in neurotransmitters and brain connectivity, similar to "rebooting" the brain.

- **Nurse's Role:** Extensive involvement:

  - **Pre-ECT:** Patient education (procedure, side effects like headache, nausea, temporary memory loss/confusion), ensure informed consent, NPO status, baseline vital signs/assessment, remove dentures/glasses/jewelry, administer pre-procedure medications (e.g., anticholinergic to decrease secretions). Provide emotional support.

  - **During ECT:** Assist psychiatrist/anesthesiologist, monitor vital signs, ensure airway patency (oxygen, suction available), monitor seizure duration (EEG).

  - **Post-ECT:** Monitor vital signs, level of consciousness, orientation frequently until stable. Manage common side effects (headache, nausea – offer analgesics/antiemetics). Reorient patient frequently (confusion/memory impairment common immediately after). Provide reassurance. Document procedure and patient response.

Transcranial Magnetic Stimulation (TMS):

- **What it is:** Uses focused magnetic pulses, delivered through a coil placed on the scalp, to stimulate specific areas of the brain (usually the prefrontal cortex for depression). Non-invasive procedure, patient is awake, no anesthesia needed. Treatments typically given daily for 4-6 weeks.

- **Uses:** Approved for Major Depressive Disorder, particularly for those who haven't responded adequately to antidepressant medication. Being explored for other conditions (OCD, anxiety). Generally less effective than ECT for severe/psychotic depression but has fewer cognitive side effects.

- **Mechanism:** Thought to modulate activity in targeted brain circuits involved in mood regulation.

- **Nurse's Role:**
    - **Patient Education:** Explain procedure, duration, potential side effects (scalp discomfort, headache, muscle twitching during pulse – generally mild).
    - **Preparation:** Ensure patient has removed any metal objects from head/neck. Position patient correctly in TMS chair.
    - **During Procedure:** Place coil accurately (per provider determination), monitor patient comfort, provide support.
    - **Post-Procedure:** Assess for side effects. Patient can usually resume normal activities immediately.
    - **Monitor Treatment Response:** Assess mood symptoms over the course of treatment.

Complementary and Alternative Therapies CAM

Many patients use therapies outside of conventional medicine, either alongside (complementary) or instead of (alternative) standard treatments. The evidence base for CAM varies greatly.

Common Examples:

- **Mind-Body Practices:** Yoga, tai chi, mindfulness meditation, biofeedback. Good evidence for stress reduction, some benefit for anxiety/depression.

- **Biologically Based:** Herbal supplements (St. John's Wort for depression – **major interaction risks!**; Kava for anxiety – liver toxicity risk; Omega-3 fatty acids – some evidence for mood), vitamins, special diets. **Safety and interactions are key concerns.**

- **Manipulative/Body-Based:** Massage therapy, acupuncture, chiropractic. May help with stress, anxiety, somatic complaints.

- **Energy Therapies:** Reiki, therapeutic touch. Less scientific evidence.

Nurse's Role:

- **Assess Use:** Routinely ask patients about *all* therapies they are using, including herbs, supplements, vitamins, and CAM practices. Many patients don't volunteer this information.

- **Educate on Safety & Interactions: Crucial!** Many CAM therapies, especially herbs/supplements, can interact dangerously with prescribed psychiatric medications (e.g., St. John's Wort + SSRI = Serotonin Syndrome risk). Provide factual information about known risks and lack of regulation for supplements.

- **Encourage Communication with Provider:** Urge patients to discuss all CAM use with their psychiatrist/primary care provider.

- **Support Evidence-Based CAM:** Encourage practices with good evidence for mental health benefits (e.g., exercise, mindfulness, yoga) as part of a holistic plan *if* the patient is interested.

- **Maintain Open, Non-Judgmental Stance:** Dismissing CAM use can shut down communication. Focus on safety and informed decision-making.

Broadening the Therapeutic Toolkit

Effective mental health care rarely relies on a single approach. Medications address biology, psychotherapies reshape thoughts and behaviors, groups provide support and social learning, brain stimulation offers options for severe conditions, and CAM therapies reflect a holistic view. The nurse, positioned centrally, needs a working knowledge of these diverse modalities—not to practice them all, but to educate patients, reinforce therapeutic work, monitor responses, ensure safety (especially with ECT and CAM interactions), and contribute meaningfully to a truly integrated, patient-centered plan of care. Understanding *what* we do brings us to *how* we organize it: the nursing process.

Core Learnings from This Section

- Psychosocial treatments are essential complements to medication.

- **Psychotherapy** involves exploring issues with a therapist. **CBT** focuses on thoughts/behaviors; **DBT** focuses on acceptance/change skills (Mindfulness,

Distress Tolerance, Emotion Regulation, Interpersonal Effectiveness). Nurse's role: Reinforce skills, support therapy goals.

- **Group Therapy** uses group dynamics for support/learning. Types: Psychoeducational, Skills, Support, Process. Nurse's role: Lead/co-lead some groups, encourage attendance, process experience.

- **ECT** is brain stimulation (induced seizure) for severe depression/mania. Nurse's role: Extensive pre-/during/post-procedure care, monitoring, education.

- **TMS** is non-invasive magnetic brain stimulation for depression. Nurse's role: Education, monitoring during procedure.

- **CAM** therapies are used alongside/instead of conventional treatment. Nurse's role: Assess use, **educate on safety/interactions (critical!)**, support evidence-based CAM, encourage provider communication.

Chapter 16:The Nursing Process in Mental Health Care

We've talked about core concepts, specific disorders, medications, and other therapies. Now, how do we put it all together systematically to provide effective, individualized care? The answer lies in the **Nursing Process**—a deliberate, problem-solving framework used across all nursing specialties, but applied here with a particular focus on the psychosocial, emotional, and behavioral needs of individuals with mental health conditions. It's not just a list of steps; it's a way of thinking critically and acting purposefully. The familiar acronym **ADPIE** guides us: Assessment, Diagnosis, Planning, Implementation, and Evaluation.

Applying ADPIE The Framework in Action

Let's walk through how each phase applies specifically in mental health nursing:

1. **Assessment:** This is the foundation. It's the ongoing process of gathering comprehensive information about the patient.

   o **Data Sources:**

      ▪ **Patient Interview:** The primary source! Using therapeutic communication skills is key. Obtain psychosocial history (family, social support, education, occupation, coping patterns, substance use, trauma history, cultural/spiritual beliefs). Assess current problems, stressors, goals.

      ▪ **Observation:** Paying close attention to behavior, appearance, speech, affect, interactions (as detailed in the MSE section).

- **Mental Status Examination (MSE):** Systematic assessment of current mental functioning.

- **Risk Assessment:** Evaluating risk of harm to self (suicide/self-harm) or others (aggression).

- **Physical Health Assessment:** Ruling out medical causes for psychiatric symptoms, assessing impact of mental illness on physical health (and vice versa), monitoring medication side effects. Vital signs, review of systems, relevant labs/diagnostics.

- **Family/Collateral Information:** Obtaining information from family or previous providers (with patient consent) can provide valuable context.

- **Records Review:** Past psychiatric history, medical history.

  - **Key Focus:** Identify not just problems, but also **strengths, resources, and coping skills** the patient possesses. This is essential for recovery-oriented care. Assessment is **continuous**, not just a one-time event.

2. **Diagnosis (Nursing Diagnosis):** This involves analyzing the assessment data to identify the patient's **responses** to actual or potential health problems that nurses can address.

   - **Use Standardized Language:** NANDA-International (NANDA-I) provides standardized nursing diagnostic labels.

- **Distinguish from Medical Diagnosis:** A medical diagnosis (e.g., Schizophrenia, MDD) identifies the disease. A nursing diagnosis identifies the related human response (e.g., *Disturbed Thought Processes*, *Risk for Suicide*, *Ineffective Coping*, *Social Isolation* related to the medical diagnosis or situation).

- **Format:** Typically includes the **Problem** (NANDA label), **Etiology** ("Related to..." factors contributing to the problem), and **Defining Characteristics** ("As evidenced by..." objective/subjective signs and symptoms from your assessment). For "Risk" diagnoses, you list risk factors instead of defining characteristics.

- **Prioritize:** Based on safety needs first (e.g., *Risk for Suicide* takes precedence over *Knowledge Deficit*). Maslow's hierarchy can be helpful (physiological/safety needs first).

3. **Planning:** This phase involves setting priorities, formulating patient-centered goals and outcomes, and selecting nursing interventions.

- **Prioritize Nursing Diagnoses:** Based on safety and patient needs.

- **Develop Goals/Outcomes:** These should be **SMART**:

  - Specific: Clearly state what should change.

  - Measurable: How will you know it's achieved? (Observable behavior, patient report, rating scale).

- **Achievable/Realistic:** Patient must be capable of reaching it with available resources/time.

- **Relevant:** Aligned with patient's overall needs and goals.

- **Time-limited:** Specify a timeframe (short-term or long-term).

- **Collaborate with Patient:** Involve the patient in goal setting whenever possible to promote buy-in and empowerment (Recovery Model principle).

- **Select Nursing Interventions:** Choose actions designed to help the patient achieve the goals. Interventions should be evidence-based, individualized, and address the etiology ("Related to" factors) of the nursing diagnosis. They cover the full scope of nursing practice (assessment, communication, education, medication, milieu, etc.).

4. **Implementation:** Putting the plan into action. This is the "doing" phase.

- **Perform Interventions:** Carry out the selected nursing actions safely and competently.

- **Coordinate Care:** Work with the interprofessional team (doctors, therapists, social workers).

- **Delegate Appropriately:** Assign tasks to other team members (e.g., mental health technicians) based on scope of practice, ensuring proper supervision.

- o **Document Actions:** Record all interventions performed and the patient's immediate response. Documentation should be timely, accurate, and objective.

5. **Evaluation:** Assessing the patient's progress toward achieving the goals and outcomes, and determining the effectiveness of the nursing interventions.

    - o **Compare Patient Response to Outcomes:** Did the patient meet the measurable criteria set in the planning phase? Fully? Partially? Not at all?

    - o **Gather Evaluation Data:** Reassess the patient (observe, interview), review documentation.

    - o **Analyze Findings:** Were the interventions effective? Why or why not? Were the goals realistic? Was the diagnosis accurate?

    - o **Modify the Care Plan:** Based on the evaluation, revise diagnoses, goals, outcomes, or interventions as needed. If goals met, determine if new goals are needed or if the problem is resolved. If not met, reassess and adjust the plan. Evaluation is ongoing and feeds back into the assessment phase, making the process cyclical.

Writing Concise and Relevant Nursing Diagnoses

A well-written nursing diagnosis accurately reflects the patient's situation and guides intervention selection. Using the NANDA-I structure helps ensure clarity and consistency.

Structure:

- **Problem:** The NANDA-I diagnostic label (e.g., *Anxiety, Risk for Suicide, Disturbed Thought Processes*).

- **Etiology:** The "Related to" (R/T) clause – identifies factors contributing to the problem (e.g., R/T perceived threat, R/T feelings of hopelessness, R/T biochemical imbalances). Should be something nurses can address through interventions. Avoid using medical diagnoses here unless linking symptoms (e.g., R/T effects of schizophrenia on thinking).

- **Defining Characteristics:** The "As Evidenced By" (AEB) clause – lists the objective and subjective data (signs/symptoms) from your assessment that support the diagnosis (e.g., AEB patient reports feeling worried, pacing, elevated heart rate; AEB patient states "Life isn't worth living," history of attempts; AEB auditory hallucinations, loose associations, poor concentration).

- **Risk Diagnoses:** Have only two parts: Problem (NANDA label starting with "Risk for...") and Risk Factors (factors increasing vulnerability, replace AEB). Example: *Risk for Self-Directed Violence* R/T history of suicide attempts, recent loss of spouse, statements of hopelessness, access to lethal means.

Common Mental Health Nursing Diagnoses List (Examples):

- Risk for Suicide

- Risk for Other-Directed Violence

- Risk for Self-Mutilation

- Ineffective Coping

- Anxiety

- Fear

- Hopelessness

- Powerlessness

222

- Spiritual Distress

- Disturbed Thought Processes

- Disturbed Sensory Perception (specify type: Auditory, Visual, etc.)

- Impaired Social Interaction

- Social Isolation

- Self-Care Deficit (specify: Bathing, Dressing, Feeding, Toileting)

- Disturbed Sleep Pattern

- Imbalanced Nutrition: Less Than Body Requirements

- Chronic Low Self-Esteem

- Ineffective Health Maintenance

- Noncompliance (use cautiously; explore reasons first)

Choose the most specific and accurate diagnosis based on your cluster of assessment data.

Developing Realistic Goals and Outcomes

Goals represent the desired change in the patient's condition or behavior. Outcomes are the specific, measurable steps towards achieving that goal. Remember **SMART**.

- **Goal (Broad Aim):** Patient will experience reduced anxiety.

  - **Outcome (Specific, Measurable):** Patient will identify 2 triggers for anxiety by end of shift.

  - **Outcome:** Patient will rate anxiety as < 4/10 using 0-10 scale by end of day.

- o **Outcome:** Patient will demonstrate one relaxation technique effectively before discharge.

- **Goal:** Patient will remain safe from self-harm.

  - o **Outcome:** Patient will state they have no intent to harm self when asked each shift.

  - o **Outcome:** Patient will contract for safety with staff (if appropriate).

  - o **Outcome:** Patient will identify one reason for living by end of week.

- **Goal:** Patient will demonstrate improved reality testing.

  - o **Outcome:** Patient will state they understand the voices are part of their illness by discharge.

  - o **Outcome:** Patient will engage in reality-based conversation for 10 minutes with staff twice per day.

Involve the patient in setting these whenever feasible. Small, achievable steps build confidence.

Selecting Appropriate Nursing Interventions

Interventions are the actions nurses take to help patients achieve their goals. They should be individualized and directly address the etiology (R/T factors) of the nursing diagnosis.

- **For *Anxiety* R/T perceived threat:**

  - o Assess anxiety level using scale.

  - o Maintain calm environment.

  - o Use therapeutic communication (active listening, validation).

- Teach relaxation techniques (deep breathing, guided imagery).
- Help patient identify triggers and coping skills.
- Administer anxiolytic medication as ordered/PRN; monitor effects.
- Educate about anxiety management.

- **For *Risk for Suicide* R/T hopelessness:**
  - Implement safety precautions (e.g., 1:1 observation, remove hazards).
  - Assess ideation/plan/intent frequently (each shift and PRN).
  - Build therapeutic rapport; convey hope.
  - Encourage expression of feelings.
  - Help patient identify reasons for living, strengths.
  - Administer antidepressants as ordered; monitor closely (esp. early treatment).
  - Develop safety plan with patient before discharge.

- **For *Disturbed Thought Processes* R/T biochemical imbalance (schizophrenia):**
  - Assess mental status, observe for hallucinations/delusions.
  - Maintain safe, structured environment.
  - Use clear, concrete communication. Avoid abstractions.
  - Gently present reality; do not argue with delusions. Validate underlying feelings.

- Administer antipsychotic medication as ordered; monitor effects/side effects (EPS, metabolic).

- Focus on reality-based activities. Redirect from delusional content.

- Educate patient/family about illness and medication adherence.

Interventions span assessment, direct care, communication, education, medication management, milieu therapy, and coordination with the team.

Documentation Tips Essential Communication

Clear, accurate, and timely documentation is critical for communication, continuity of care, legal protection, and quality improvement.

- **Be Objective:** Describe what you see, hear, and do. Use behavioral descriptions ("Patient pacing hall, clenched fists") instead of interpretations ("Patient agitated and angry").

- **Use Quotes:** Record significant patient statements verbatim.

- **Be Concise but Complete:** Include relevant details but avoid unnecessary jargon or rambling.

- **Document the Nursing Process:** Show evidence of assessment findings, nursing diagnoses addressed, interventions performed, and patient's response (evaluation). Focus notes (DAR - Data, Action, Response) or SOAP notes can structure this.

- **Document Changes:** Note any changes (improvement or decline) in patient's condition, behavior, or mental status.

- **Document Safety:** Thoroughly record all risk assessments (suicide, violence), safety precautions implemented, and patient responses.

- **Document Education:** Note what was taught, patient/family understanding (use teach-back), and any materials provided.

- **Document Non-Adherence/Refusals:** Record if patient refuses medication or treatment, your actions (e.g., education provided, provider notified), and the patient's stated reason if given.

- **Timeliness:** Document as close to the time of assessment or intervention as possible. Late entries require clear notation.

- **Legibility/Accuracy:** Ensure entries are legible (if handwritten), accurate, and signed correctly with date/time/credentials. Follow institutional policies for electronic health records.

Sample Care Plan Snippets (Text Description):

- **Scenario 1: Anxiety**

  - *Nsg Dx:* Anxiety R/T upcoming court date AEB patient reports "constant worry," pacing, hand-wringing, states "I can't sleep."

  - *Goal/Outcome:* Patient will report reduced anxiety level by end of shift. Patient will rate anxiety < 5/10.

  - *Interventions:* Assess anxiety q4h using scale. Encourage verbalization of fears. Teach deep breathing technique. Offer PRN lorazepam as ordered for severe anxiety. Reduce environmental stimuli.

- ○ *Evaluation:* Patient practiced deep breathing, accepted PRN med. Reported anxiety 6/10 at end of shift. Goal partially met. Continue plan, reinforce coping skills.

- **Scenario 2: Risk for Self-Directed Violence**

  - ○ *Nsg Dx:* Risk for Self-Directed Violence R/T command hallucinations urging self-harm, history of attempts.

  - ○ *Goal/Outcome:* Patient will remain safe and free from self-harm during shift.

  - ○ *Interventions:* Institute 1:1 constant observation. Assess for hallucinations/SI q1h and PRN. Remove potentially dangerous items from room/patient possession. Build rapport, encourage reporting of voices. Administer antipsychotic as ordered.

  - ○ *Evaluation:* Patient remained safe, no self-harm attempts. Reported continued voices but denied intent to act on them. Goal met. Continue 1:1 observation and plan.

The Nurse's Compass

The nursing process is more than just paperwork; it's the intellectual engine driving professional nursing practice. In mental health, it guides us through complex human experiences, helping us move from simply observing symptoms to understanding responses, planning thoughtful interventions, and evaluating their impact. It ensures our care is organized, individualized, goal-directed, and—most importantly—centered on the patient's unique needs and journey toward recovery. It is our compass in navigating the often-challenging terrain of mental health care. Now, let's focus on managing acute situations where that navigation becomes critical: crisis intervention and de-escalation.

Core Learnings from This Section

- The **Nursing Process (ADPIE)** provides a systematic framework for mental health nursing care.

- **Assessment:** Ongoing gathering of subjective/objective data (MSE, risk, physical health, strengths).

- **Diagnosis (Nursing):** Identifies patient responses (Problem R/T Etiology AEB Defining Characteristics). Prioritize safety.

- **Planning:** Setting **SMART** goals/outcomes collaboratively with patient; selecting interventions.

- **Implementation:** Performing interventions (communication, meds, education, milieu); documenting actions.

- **Evaluation:** Assessing progress toward goals; modifying plan as needed. Cyclical process.

- **Documentation** must be objective, concise, timely, and reflect the nursing process.

Chapter 17: Crisis Intervention and De-escalation Techniques

Moments of crisis are inevitable in mental health settings—and indeed, across all healthcare environments. A **crisis** occurs when a person faces a situation they perceive as overwhelming, and their usual coping mechanisms fail, leading to acute distress, disorganization, and potential danger to self or others. While crises are challenging, they also represent turning points. Effective **crisis intervention** aims to provide immediate support to stabilize the situation, ensure safety, reduce distress, and help the person regain equilibrium and access coping resources. A key skill within this is **de-escalation**—verbally and non-verbally calming a potentially agitated or aggressive individual to prevent harm.

Recognizing Escalating Behavior

The earlier you can recognize signs of escalating agitation or anger, the better your chances of intervening successfully before the situation becomes dangerous. Prevention and early detection are paramount. Watch for clusters of behaviors, changes from baseline, and consider context.

Potential Warning Signs (Verbal and Nonverbal):

- **Verbal Cues:**
    - **Volume:** Loud, shouting.
    - **Tone:** Angry, hostile, sarcastic, demanding.
    - **Content:** Swearing, threatening language ("You'll be sorry," "I'll hurt you/myself"), refusing requests, making personal insults, challenging staff.
    - **Pace:** Rapid, pressured speech.

- **Nonverbal Cues (Body Language):**

    o **Motor Activity:** Pacing, restlessness, agitation, inability to sit still, pounding fists, kicking objects, throwing things.

    o **Posture:** Rigid, tense, leaning forward aggressively, clenched jaw/fists.

    o **Personal Space:** Invading others' space or your own.

    o **Eyes:** Intense staring, glaring, dilated pupils, avoidance of eye contact (can signal fear/feeling cornered).

    o **Facial Expression:** Angry, flushed face, frowning.

- **Other Signs:**

    o Sudden change in behavior from baseline.

    o Confusion or disorientation (can lead to fear/agitation).

    o Signs of substance intoxication or withdrawal.

    o History of violence or impulsivity (use caution, don't assume, but be aware).

Trust your instincts. If a situation feels tense or unsafe, it probably is. Don't ignore warning signs.

Verbal and Non verbal De escalation Strategies

The goal of de-escalation is to use communication and environmental management to reduce the intensity of a situation without resorting to physical interventions. It requires calmness, confidence, and specific techniques.

Non-Verbal Strategies (Your Body Language & Positioning):

1. **Maintain Calm Demeanor:** Control your own breathing, appear calm and self-assured (even if you feel anxious). Your calmness can be contagious. Avoid showing fear or anger.

2. **Respect Personal Space:** Stand at least 1.5 to 3 feet away (or further if needed). Don't crowd the person. Standing at an angle (not directly face-to-face) can feel less confrontational.

3. **Keep Hands Visible & Relaxed:** Avoid clenched fists, crossed arms, or hands in pockets. Keep hands open and below your waist.

4. **Use Neutral Facial Expression:** Avoid smiling (can seem mocking) or frowning (can seem challenging). Aim for concerned neutrality.

5. **Limit Eye Contact:** Avoid intense staring, which can feel threatening. Use intermittent, natural eye contact.

6. **Position for Safety:** Stand near an exit but do not block the patient's exit route (unless necessary for safety of others). Avoid letting the agitated person get between you and the door. Never turn your back.

Verbal Strategies (What You Say & How You Say It):

1. **Use Calm Tone & Volume:** Speak slowly, clearly, and quietly or at a normal volume. Lowering your voice can sometimes encourage the other person to lower theirs.

2. **Listen Actively:** Allow the person to vent (within limits). Use active listening skills (nodding, brief encouragers) to show you are hearing their concerns, even if irrational. Try to understand the *feeling* behind the words.

3. **Validate Feelings (Not Behavior):** Acknowledge their emotional state without condoning aggression. "I can

see you're very upset right now." "It sounds like you feel angry about [the situation]." Avoid minimizing ("Calm down," "It's not a big deal").

4. **Use Simple, Clear Language:** Avoid jargon, complex sentences, or abstract concepts. Especially important if the person is confused or psychotic.

5. **Be Respectful:** Use polite language ("Mr. Jones," "please," "thank you"). Avoid sarcasm, threats, or insults.

6. **Focus on the Here and Now:** Bring the conversation back to the current situation and how to resolve it peacefully. Avoid dwelling on past grievances during acute agitation.

7. **Offer Choices & Options:** Give the person a sense of control over small things. "Would you prefer to talk about this here, or would it be better to go to the quiet room?" "Would you like to try taking some deep breaths, or would taking your PRN medication be more helpful right now?" (Only offer options you can actually follow through on).

8. **Set Clear, Consistent Limits:** If behavior is unacceptable (e.g., threats, intense yelling), state the limit calmly and firmly, focusing on the behavior. "Shouting makes it difficult to understand you. We need to speak more calmly." "Threatening language is not acceptable here." Explain consequences simply if limits are not respected.

9. **Know When to Stop Talking:** Sometimes silence, allowing the person time to process, is more effective than continuous talking.

10. **Suggest Alternatives:** Offer constructive ways to express anger or frustration (e.g., talking it out, physical exercise later, using coping skills).

De-escalation Step-by-Step Guide (Conceptual Flow):

1. **Assess:** Quickly assess the situation, level of agitation, potential risks, presence of others, environmental hazards. Ensure your own safety first (positioning, backup nearby).

2. **Engage Respectfully:** Approach calmly, introduce self if needed, use person's name.

3. **Listen Actively:** Allow venting (briefly), identify core issue/feeling if possible.

4. **Validate Feelings:** Acknowledge their emotional state non-judgmentally.

5. **Set Limits (if needed):** Calmly address unsafe/unacceptable behavior.

6. **Offer Choices/Solutions:** Propose ways to resolve the immediate issue or manage distress (talking, meds, quiet space, coping skill).

7. **Negotiate (if appropriate):** Work towards a mutually acceptable resolution if feasible.

8. **Disengage (if escalating/unsafe):** Know when to back away and call for help. State clearly you are leaving to get assistance if needed.

Managing Agitation and Aggression Safely

Sometimes, despite best efforts, verbal de-escalation fails, and the risk of physical aggression becomes imminent. Managing this requires a team approach prioritizing safety for everyone.

Key Principles:

234

1. **Safety First:** Protect yourself, other patients, and the agitated individual. Remove potential weapons (objects that can be thrown or used to hit). Ensure adequate space.

2. **Call for Help:** Never attempt to manage physical aggression alone. Use the facility's emergency code system or call for backup immediately. A coordinated team response is essential.

3. **Team Approach:** Have enough trained staff present (often 4-5 people minimum for physical restraint). Designate a team leader to direct the intervention clearly and calmly.

4. **Show of Support:** The visible presence of several calm, confident staff members can sometimes deter physical aggression without needing hands-on intervention.

5. **Offer Medication:** Clearly offer PRN medication (oral liquid concentrate often preferred for speed/less coercion; IM as next option if refused/unsafe) to help the patient regain control. Frame it as help, not punishment. "This medication can help you feel calmer and more in control."

6. **Maintain Calm Communication:** Even if preparing for physical intervention, the team leader should continue trying to communicate calmly with the patient.

7. **Physical Intervention (Restraint) as Last Resort:** Only if imminent risk of harm exists and less restrictive measures have failed. Requires specific training (e.g., CPI, MANDT). Use minimum force necessary. Ensure patient/staff safety during the hold. Follow facility protocol meticulously.

Understanding Seclusion and Restraints

Seclusion (involuntary confinement alone) and restraints (manual holds or mechanical devices limiting movement) are highly restrictive interventions used **only** in emergencies to prevent imminent harm when less restrictive methods are ineffective. Their use is heavily regulated and requires strict adherence to protocols and patient rights.

Key Points:

- **LAST RESORT:** Absolutely only when immediate physical safety is at risk. Cannot be used for punishment, coercion, convenience, or as a substitute for adequate staffing/treatment.

- **Imminent Danger:** Clear risk of harm to self or others *right now*.

- **Order Required:** Must have a physician's or licensed independent practitioner's order obtained promptly (can be initiated by RN in true emergency, followed immediately by obtaining order per facility policy). Order must specify type, reason, duration (time-limited, usually 1-4 hours depending on age/policy). Re-evaluation and new orders needed for continuation.

- **Least Restrictive:** Must try less restrictive measures first (verbal de-escalation, medication offer, reducing stimuli, 1:1 observation). Document what was tried and failed.

- **Continuous Monitoring:** Usually requires constant face-to-face observation or video monitoring with frequent checks by RN. Assess vital signs, circulation (if mechanical restraints), hydration, nutrition, toileting needs, skin integrity, psychological state, readiness for release.

- **Documentation:** Meticulous documentation is required: reason for use, less restrictive measures tried, type/time applied, patient behavior, all assessments/care provided during use, time discontinued, patient response upon release.

- **Patient Rights:** Patients still have rights during seclusion/restraint (e.g., right to be informed, right to have needs met).

- **Debriefing:** Essential afterward for both the patient (explore triggers, alternatives) and staff (review event, identify learning opportunities, manage staff stress).

Safety Protocol Reminders:

- Always be aware of your surroundings and potential exits.

- Know your facility's emergency codes and procedures.

- Remove potential weapons from the environment (and yourself - e.g., dangling necklaces, ties).

- Attempt de-escalation but don't put yourself in danger; call for help early.

- Work as a team; communicate clearly during interventions.

- Never manage physical aggression alone.

- Follow seclusion/restraint protocols precisely.

- Document everything thoroughly.

Maintaining Calm in the Storm

Crises and escalation are high-stress situations for everyone involved. The ability to remain calm, think clearly, and apply de-escalation techniques effectively is a learned skill, honed through practice, training, and self-reflection. Prioritizing safety—for the patient, yourself, and others—is always the guiding principle. Recognizing warning signs early, intervening respectfully, using verbal and non-verbal skills strategically, working as a team, and using restrictive interventions only as a true last resort are hallmarks of professional crisis management in mental health nursing.

Core Learnings from This Section

- **Crisis:** Acute disruption where coping fails. **Crisis Intervention:** Immediate support to stabilize, ensure safety, restore equilibrium.

- **Recognize Escalation:** Watch for verbal (loud, threats) and nonverbal (pacing, clenched fists, rigid posture) warning signs. Early detection is key.

- **De-escalation:** Use **Non-verbal** skills (calm presence, personal space, open posture) and **Verbal** skills (calm tone, active listening, validation, offering choices, setting limits) to reduce agitation.

- **Manage Aggression Safely:** Prioritize safety, call for help (team approach), offer medication, use seclusion/restraint **only as a last resort** for imminent danger.

- **Seclusion/Restraint:** Requires order, strict monitoring, documentation, adherence to patient rights, debriefing. Not for punishment/convenience.

- Safety protocols (awareness, backup, team communication) are essential.

Part 4: Special Topics & Professional Issues

Chapter 18 Legal and Ethical Considerations

Mental health nursing doesn't happen in a vacuum. We practice within a complex web of laws, regulations, and ethical principles designed to protect the rights and safety of a vulnerable population while ensuring appropriate care can be delivered. Navigating this requires knowledge, careful judgment, and a strong ethical compass. Understanding patient rights, the conditions under which treatment can be compelled, our duty regarding confidentiality, and how to approach ethical quandaries are all essential aspects of safe, responsible nursing practice.

Patient Rights Keeping Patients at the Center

Individuals receiving mental health care—even those hospitalized involuntarily—retain fundamental rights. Upholding these rights is not just a legal requirement; it's central to building trust and promoting recovery. Key rights include:

- **The Right to Treatment:** Patients have the right to receive appropriate medical and psychiatric care. This includes having an individualized treatment plan and having that plan reviewed and updated regularly. Care should be provided in the **Least Restrictive Environment** possible—meaning treatment should occur in settings that allow the greatest freedom consistent with the patient's safety and treatment needs (e.g., outpatient before inpatient, unlocked unit before locked unit, verbal de-escalation before seclusion/restraint).

- **The Right to Refuse Treatment (Including Medication):** This is a cornerstone of patient autonomy. Generally, **competent** adults have the right to refuse any treatment, including psychotropic medications.

  - **Competency:** This is a legal determination (not just clinical judgment) that a person has the capacity to understand information about their condition and proposed treatment (including risks, benefits, alternatives) and to make a reasoned decision. Mental illness does *not* automatically mean incompetence.

- **Exceptions:** The right to refuse can be overridden under specific circumstances, varying by jurisdiction, but typically involving:

  1. **Emergencies:** When immediate treatment is needed to prevent serious harm to self or others, medication might be given without consent.

  2. **Incompetency:** If a patient is legally determined incompetent to make treatment decisions, a guardian or surrogate decision-maker may consent, or treatment may be court-ordered.

  3. **Court Orders:** Specific court orders can mandate outpatient treatment (Assisted Outpatient Treatment - AOT) or inpatient treatment, including medication, if strict criteria regarding danger/disability are met.

- **Nurse's Role:** Educate patients about proposed treatments, assess understanding, explore reasons for refusal non-judgmentally, document refusal and actions taken, advocate for the patient's wishes when appropriate, and administer treatment safely when legally authorized (e.g., via court order or emergency protocol). Never coerce or trick patients into taking medication.

- **The Right to Informed Consent:** Before any non-emergency treatment, patients have the right to receive adequate information to make an informed decision. This includes: the nature of their condition, the purpose of the proposed treatment, potential risks and benefits, alternative treatments (including no treatment), and the right to withdraw consent. Consent must be voluntary and given by a competent individual.

- **Confidentiality:** Patients have a right to have information about their condition and treatment kept private. This is protected by ethical codes and laws (like HIPAA in the United States). Information should only be shared with others involved in the patient's direct care on a need-to-know basis, or with specific patient authorization.

  - **Limits to Confidentiality:** Explain these clearly upfront. Exceptions include:

    - **Duty to Warn:** If a patient makes specific threats against an identifiable person (see below).

    - **Suspected Abuse/Neglect:** Mandated reporting laws require reporting suspected abuse or neglect of children, elders, or vulnerable adults.

    - **Court Orders/Legal Proceedings:** Information may be required by subpoena or court order.

- **Other Important Rights:** Include the right to humane treatment, dignity, respect, freedom from abuse and neglect, communication (access to mail, phone, visitors - within safety limits), privacy, keeping personal possessions (if safe), lodging complaints or grievances without reprisal, and access to legal counsel or patient advocates.

Case Snippet: Right to Refuse

- *Scenario:* Mr. Green, admitted voluntarily for depression, refuses his prescribed antidepressant, stating, "I read online it causes weight gain, and I don't want that." He appears to understand the medication's purpose and alternatives explained by the physician. He shows no signs of imminent danger to self or others.

- *Nursing Considerations:* Mr. Green is voluntary and appears competent to refuse. The nurse should: Acknowledge his concern ("I understand you're worried about potential weight gain"), explore his understanding further, reinforce education about risks/benefits/alternatives, document his refusal and the reason given, notify the prescriber, and continue to provide other supportive nursing care. Forcing the medication would violate his rights. The team may need to explore alternative medications or treatment strategies.

Involuntary Commitment Basics When Treatment Is Mandated

While most mental health treatment is voluntary, sometimes individuals are hospitalized or treated against their will. **Involuntary commitment** (also called civil commitment) is a legal process, governed by state/jurisdictional laws, allowing for temporary detention and treatment of individuals who meet specific criteria.

General Criteria (Varies by Location): Typically requires proof (often "clear and convincing evidence") that the person:

1. Has a **diagnosable mental illness**, AND

2. Poses an imminent **danger to self** (suicidal, unable to provide basic care leading to harm), OR

3. Poses an imminent **danger to others** (homicidal, assaultive), OR

4. Is **gravely disabled** (unable to provide for basic needs like food, clothing, shelter due to mental illness, leading to likely harm).

Process Overview (Simplified & General):

1. **Initial Hold/Detention:** Often begins with an emergency hold (e.g., 48-72 hours) initiated by police, physician, or designated mental health professional based on probable cause meeting criteria. Allows for evaluation.

2. **Evaluation:** Psychiatrists and other professionals assess the patient to determine if commitment criteria are met.

3. **Court Hearing:** If longer commitment is sought, a formal court hearing occurs. The patient has legal rights, including notice of the hearing, right to legal counsel (often court-appointed), right to be present, right to present evidence and cross-examine witnesses.

4. **Commitment Order:** If the court finds criteria are met, it issues an order for a specific period of inpatient or outpatient treatment. This order may include authorization for medication over objection if specific criteria regarding incompetency/danger are also met.

5. **Periodic Review:** Commitment orders are time-limited and require regular review by the court to determine if criteria for continued commitment are still met.

Important Points:

- Involuntary commitment is a **legal**, not just clinical, process.Strict procedures must be followed.

- Patients under commitment **still retain most civil rights**, including the right to quality treatment, confidentiality (with exceptions), communication, etc. They lose the right to leave the facility freely.

- The **right to refuse medication** may be overridden by court order or in emergencies, but this requires specific justification beyond the commitment itself.

Nurse's Role: Careful assessment documenting behaviors supporting commitment criteria (danger, disability), providing safe care, educating patient/family about the process and their rights, administering treatment as legally authorized, advocating for least restrictive setting, testifying at hearings if required.

Duty to Warn Protecting Potential Victims

This is a significant exception to patient confidentiality. Stemming from the landmark *Tarasoff v. Regents of University of California* case, it establishes that mental health professionals have a duty to protect third parties from potential harm by a patient.

Key Elements:

1. Patient communicates a **serious threat** of physical violence.

2. Threat is against a **reasonably identifiable victim(s)**.

3. There is a **foreseeable risk** of harm.

If these conditions are met, the clinician has a duty to take reasonable steps to protect the potential victim. This may involve:

- Warning the potential victim directly.

- Notifying law enforcement.

- Taking steps to have the patient hospitalized (if commitment criteria met).

Nurse's Role: If a patient makes such a threat, the nurse must take it seriously. Assess the seriousness, specificity, and imminence of the threat. **Immediately report the threat to the treatment team leader and supervisor.** Follow facility policy precisely. Documentation is critical. Do *not* try to handle this alone. The decision on *how* to fulfill the duty (warn victim, call police) is typically made by the treatment team/provider after careful consideration.

Case Snippet: Duty to Warn

- *Scenario:* During a therapy session on an inpatient unit, a patient, Mr. Vance, tells his nurse, "When I get out of here, I'm going straight to my ex-wife Linda's house, and she's going to pay for leaving me. I know where she lives." He appears angry and intense.

- *Nursing Considerations:* This constitutes a specific threat against an identifiable victim. The nurse must: Immediately inform the psychiatrist and treatment team. Document Mr. Vance's statement verbatim, his affect, and the notification of the team. The team will then assess the risk and determine the appropriate steps (e.g., further risk assessment, possibly initiating commitment proceedings if he meets criteria, contacting law enforcement, and/or contacting Linda to warn her, depending on local laws and team judgment). The nurse supports the team's plan and continues to monitor Mr. Vance.

Ethical Dilemmas in Mental Health Nursing Navigating Gray Areas

Sometimes, legal rules are clear, but ethical situations are murky. An **ethical dilemma** arises when there is a conflict between two or more ethical principles (e.g., patient autonomy vs. beneficence - doing good) or professional values. Mental health nursing is ripe with potential dilemmas.

Common Examples:

- **Forced Medication:** Balancing the patient's right to refuse (autonomy) against the need to treat severe symptoms causing suffering or danger (beneficence, non-maleficence - do no harm). When is overriding refusal ethically justifiable?

- **Confidentiality vs. Safety:** Deciding when potential harm (to self, others, or due to abuse) outweighs the duty of confidentiality. How serious must the risk be?

- **Resource Allocation:** How to distribute limited nursing time or resources fairly among patients with competing needs?

- **Boundary Issues:** Navigating gifts, self-disclosure, or patient requests that blur professional lines (autonomy vs. professional integrity).

- **Truth-Telling:** How much information to share with families when the patient refuses consent but family involvement could be beneficial? Balancing confidentiality with family needs/support.

- **Use of Restraints/Seclusion:** Balancing safety needs (non-maleficence) with the patient's right to freedom and dignity (autonomy, justice). Is it truly the least restrictive option?

- **Reporting Impaired Colleagues:** Duty to protect patients (non-maleficence) versus loyalty to a colleague.

Ethical Decision-Making Points A Framework:

There's no easy formula, but a structured approach helps:

1. **Identify the Dilemma:** Clearly state the conflicting ethical principles or values involved (e.g., Autonomy vs. Beneficence).

2. **Gather Information:** Collect all relevant clinical facts, patient preferences/values, legal constraints (laws, policies), professional codes (e.g., ANA Code of Ethics), and perspectives of stakeholders (patient, family, team).

3. **Examine Options:** Brainstorm possible courses of action.

4. **Analyze Consequences:** Consider the potential positive and negative outcomes of each option for all stakeholders. How does each option align with ethical principles?

5. **Choose & Act:** Select the option that seems most ethically justifiable, balancing the principles involved. Be prepared to articulate your reasoning.

6. **Evaluate:** Reflect on the outcome of the action. What was learned? Could anything have been done differently?

7. **Seek Consultation: Crucial step!** Discuss the dilemma with supervisors, experienced colleagues, the ethics committee, or mentors. Don't try to resolve complex ethical issues in isolation.

Key Legal Terms Glossary (Text Description):

- **Informed Consent:** Process of ensuring a patient understands their condition, proposed treatment (risks, benefits, alternatives), and voluntarily agrees. Requires competency.

- **Competency:** Legal term indicating a person's ability to understand information and make rational decisions regarding their care. Distinct from capacity (clinical judgment).

- **Involuntary Commitment:** Legal process allowing detention/treatment of individuals with mental illness meeting criteria (danger to self/others, gravely disabled).

- **Least Restrictive Environment:** Principle that patients should be treated in settings allowing maximal freedom consistent with safety/treatment needs.

- **Confidentiality:** Ethical and legal duty to keep patient information private, with specific exceptions.

- **HIPAA (Health Insurance Portability and Accountability Act):** US federal law protecting privacy of health information.

- **Duty to Warn (Tarasoff Duty):** Legal/ethical obligation to take steps to protect an identifiable third party from serious threats made by a patient.

Balancing Rights and Responsibilities

The legal and ethical landscape of mental health nursing is complex, requiring constant vigilance to uphold patient rights while ensuring safety and providing effective care. Knowing the specific laws in your jurisdiction is essential, as is familiarity with your professional code of ethics. When faced with dilemmas, a structured decision-making process and consultation with colleagues and supervisors are invaluable. Ultimately, our practice must be grounded in respect for patient autonomy and dignity, tempered by our professional responsibility to protect vulnerable individuals and the community. From these guiding principles, we turn to adapting our care across different ages and diverse populations.

Core Learnings from This Section

- Mental health patients retain fundamental **rights**, including treatment in the least restrictive environment, informed consent, confidentiality (with limits), and generally, the right to refuse treatment if competent.

- **Involuntary Commitment** is a legal process for treating individuals with mental illness who pose a danger to self/others or are gravely disabled; it requires strict adherence to procedures and patient rights.

- **Duty to Warn** mandates overriding confidentiality to protect identifiable victims from serious threats. Report threats to the team immediately.

- **Ethical Dilemmas** involve conflicting principles; use a structured **decision-making framework** and **seek consultation**.

- Nurses must know relevant laws, ethical codes, and facility policies to practice safely and ethically.

Chapter 19: Caring Across the Lifespan and Diverse Populations

Mental health needs, how they are expressed, and how people respond to care vary significantly across different age groups and cultural backgrounds. A one-size-fits-all approach simply doesn't work. Effective mental health nursing requires adapting our assessments, communication styles, and interventions to meet the unique needs presented by children, adolescents, older adults, and individuals from diverse cultural, ethnic, and identity groups. This demands flexibility, sensitivity, and a commitment to understanding each person within their specific context.

Key Considerations for Children and Adolescents

Working with younger populations requires a developmental perspective. What's considered normal behavior changes rapidly through childhood and adolescence.

- **Developmental Context:** Assess behavior in relation to developmental milestones. Temper tantrums are normal in toddlers but concerning in teenagers. Difficulty concentrating might be ADHD, anxiety, or a reaction to family stress—context is everything.

- **Assessment Differences:**

    - **Reliance on Collateral:** Information from parents, caregivers, and teachers is often crucial, as children may struggle to articulate internal states. Observe discrepancies between reports.

    - **Communication:** Use age-appropriate language. Engage younger children through **play, drawing, or storytelling**, which can be powerful assessment tools. Build rapport gradually. Be patient.

- o **Family System:** Problems often exist within the family context. Assessment and treatment usually need to involve the family unit. Observe family interactions.

- **Common Issues:** While children/adolescents can experience the full range of mental disorders, some are more commonly diagnosed in these age groups:

  - o **Neurodevelopmental Disorders:** ADHD (inattention, hyperactivity/impulsivity), Autism Spectrum Disorder (social communication deficits, restricted/repetitive behaviors), Intellectual Disability, Specific Learning Disorders.

  - o **Disruptive, Impulse-Control, and Conduct Disorders:** Oppositional Defiant Disorder (negativistic, defiant behavior), Conduct Disorder (violating rights of others, aggression, destruction).

  - o **Anxiety Disorders:** Separation anxiety, specific phobias, social anxiety, GAD.

  - o **Depression:** Can present differently than in adults (more irritability, somatic complaints, social withdrawal). Suicide risk is a serious concern in adolescents.

- **Treatment Approaches:**

  - o **Family Therapy:** Often a primary modality.

  - o **Play Therapy:** For younger children to express feelings/experiences non-verbally.

  - o **Parent Management Training (PMT):** Teaching parents effective behavior management techniques.

252

- **Individual Therapy:** CBT and DBT adapted for younger ages.

- **Medication:** Used cautiously, often after psychosocial interventions. Requires careful monitoring for side effects, including impact on growth and development. Stimulants for ADHD, SSRIs for depression/anxiety, antipsychotics for psychosis or severe aggression.

- **School Collaboration:** Working with school counselors/psychologists is often essential.

- **Age-Specific Communication Tips:**

  - **Young Children:** Get down on their level (physically). Use play, simple words, drawings. Be patient. Validate feelings simply.

  - **School-Age Children:** Can use more direct questions but still benefit from games or drawing. Explain things concretely. Be honest.

  - **Adolescents:** Respect their need for independence/privacy (explain confidentiality limits clearly). Avoid jargon or "talking down." Be genuine and direct. Allow them to express opinions. Be mindful of peer group importance.

Case Snippet: Adolescent Depression

- *Scenario:* Maya, 15, is brought in by her parents due to declining grades, social withdrawal (spending most time alone in her room), increased irritability, difficulty sleeping, and vague complaints of stomach aches. She tearfully tells the nurse, "Everything feels pointless."

- *Nursing Considerations:* Assess for MDD symptoms (SIGECAPS), paying attention to irritability and somatic complaints common in teens. **Prioritize suicide risk assessment.** Build rapport by listening respectfully, validating her feelings. Involve parents in assessment but also interview Maya alone (explaining confidentiality limits). Explore stressors (school, peers, family). Nursing care involves safety monitoring, encouraging participation in therapy (individual/family), medication education if prescribed, supporting healthy routines (sleep, activity), and collaborating with school if appropriate.

Key Considerations for Older Adults

Mental health care for older adults (typically 65+) requires attention to unique factors related to aging, physical health, and social circumstances.

- **Age is Not Illness:** It's critical to distinguish normal aging changes from pathological conditions. Depression, anxiety, or significant cognitive decline are **not** normal parts of aging.

- **Under-recognition:** Mental health problems are often missed or misattributed to aging or physical illness by patients, families, and even providers. Stigma may be higher in this cohort.

- **Common Issues:**

  - **Depression:** Very common, often presents with physical complaints (pain, fatigue) rather than sadness ("masked depression"). Suicide risk is particularly high in older white males. Losses (spouse, friends, health, independence) are significant risk factors.

  - **Anxiety Disorders:** Also common, may overlap with medical conditions.

- **Neurocognitive Disorders (NCDs):** Dementia (Alzheimer's most common) and Delirium (often due to medical illness/meds). Accurate differentiation is crucial (see Chapter 13).

- **Substance Use:** Often involves alcohol or misuse of prescription medications (sedatives, pain meds). Can be easily missed.

- **Sleep Disorders.**

- **Assessment Challenges:**

  - **Comorbid Medical Conditions:** Physical illnesses can cause or mimic psychiatric symptoms (e.g., thyroid issues and depression/anxiety). Symptoms can overlap.

  - **Polypharmacy:** Older adults often take multiple medications, increasing risk of side effects and drug interactions that can cause cognitive/mood changes.

  - **Sensory Deficits:** Hearing/vision loss can impact communication and assessment, potentially leading to isolation or appearing confused.

  - **Cognitive Changes:** Need to assess cognition baseline and changes carefully (using tools like Mini-Mental State Exam - MMSE or Montreal Cognitive Assessment - MoCA).

- **Communication Strategies:**

  - **Address Sensory Issues:** Ensure hearing aids/glasses are working. Speak clearly, face the person, minimize background noise. Use larger print materials.

- o **Allow More Time:** Processing speed may be slower. Avoid rushing.

- o **Be Respectful:** Avoid patronizing language or "elderspeak." Address patient formally unless invited otherwise.

- o **Focus on Concrete Issues:** Start with physical concerns if that's the patient's focus, then gently explore mood/function.

- **Treatment Considerations:**

  - o **Medication:** "Start low, go slow." Older adults metabolize drugs differently, are more sensitive to side effects (especially anticholinergic effects, sedation, orthostasis - fall risk!). Monitor closely. Polypharmacy review is essential.

  - o **Psychosocial Approaches:** Therapy (CBT, reminiscence therapy, supportive therapy) is effective. Group therapy, senior center activities can reduce isolation. Emphasis on maintaining function and quality of life.

- **Age-Specific Communication Tip (Older Adults):** Begin interview by establishing rapport, inquire about physical comfort, and clearly explain the purpose of the interaction, allowing ample time for response.

Case Snippet: Older Adult Depression

- *Scenario:* Mr. Peterson, 78, a widower living alone, sees his GP for persistent back pain and fatigue. His daughter notes he rarely leaves the house anymore, has lost weight, and seems disinterested in his usual hobbies (gardening, watching football). Mr. Peterson denies feeling "sad" but admits to poor sleep, low energy, and feeling "slowed down."

- *Nursing Considerations:* The nurse should screen for depression using a geriatric-specific tool. Priorities include exploring the link between physical symptoms and potential depression, assessing functional decline and social isolation, evaluating suicide risk (especially given age/widower status), reviewing medications for potential contribution, encouraging socialization and activity (perhaps suggesting senior center), discussing treatment options (meds started low, therapy), and involving the daughter for support (with Mr. Peterson's permission).

Cultural Humility and Culturally Competent Care

As emphasized before, culture shapes every aspect of the mental health experience. Providing effective care requires moving beyond simply knowing facts about different groups (**cultural competence**) towards **cultural humility**—a stance of openness, self-reflection, and lifelong learning.

Key Reminders:

- **Self-Reflection:** Continuously examine your own biases, assumptions, and cultural worldview. How might these influence your interactions?

- **Patient as Expert:** Approach each patient as an individual. Ask them directly about their beliefs, values, practices, and preferences related to health, illness, and help-seeking. **"What is important for me to know about you and your background to provide you with the best care?"**

- **Symptom Expression:** Recognize that distress may be expressed differently (e.g., somatically, through religious idioms). Avoid misinterpreting culturally normative behaviors as pathology.

- **Family & Community:** Understand the role of family and community in decision-making and support systems, which varies greatly across cultures.

- **Stigma:** Be sensitive to varying levels and types of stigma associated with mental illness.

- **Language Barriers: Always use qualified medical interpreters** for patients with limited English proficiency. Do NOT rely on family members (especially children), as this compromises confidentiality, accuracy, and power dynamics. Document interpreter use.

- **Treatment Preferences:** Explore patient preferences for different types of treatment (medication, therapy, traditional healing, spiritual support). Integrate these respectfully and safely whenever possible.

Cultural Sensitivity Reminders (Questions to Consider Asking):

- "How do you/your family understand this problem?"

- "What do you believe causes this kind of problem?"

- "What kind of treatments do you think might help?" (Explore traditional/alternative practices).

- "Who in your family/community usually helps make decisions about health?"

- "Is there anything about your background or beliefs that would be important for me to know?"

Caring for LGBTQ Individuals

Lesbian, Gay, Bisexual, Transgender, Queer/Questioning (LGBTQ+) individuals face unique stressors related to societal stigma, discrimination, and potential lack of acceptance, contributing to higher rates of certain mental health conditions. Providing affirming care is essential.

- **Minority Stress:** Understand the concept – chronic stress arising from stigma, prejudice, discrimination, and internalized negative societal messages.

- **Create Welcoming Environment:** Use inclusive language on forms and in conversation. Display symbols of inclusivity (e.g., rainbow flag). Ensure policies are non-discriminatory.

- **Use Correct Names & Pronouns:** Ask patients respectfully how they wish to be addressed and what pronouns they use (she/her, he/him, they/them, etc.). Use these consistently. Apologize briefly if you make a mistake and correct yourself.

- **Don't Assume:** Don't assume sexual orientation or gender identity based on appearance or relationship status. If relevant to care, ask open-ended, non-judgmental questions.

- **Be Aware of Health Disparities:** Higher rates of depression, anxiety, PTSD, substance use, suicide attempts. Understand specific stressors (coming out, family rejection, discrimination, violence, issues related to gender transition if applicable).

- **Provide Affirming Care:** Validate identity and experiences. Connect patients with LGBTQ+-affirming resources and providers if needed. Educate yourself on relevant health issues (e.g., effects of hormone therapy).

Addressing Social Determinants of Health SDOH

Mental health doesn't exist in isolation from social conditions. **Social Determinants of Health (SDOH)** are the non-medical factors significantly influencing health outcomes.

- **Key SDOH impacting Mental Health:**

- **Economic Stability:** Poverty, unemployment, housing instability, food insecurity.

- **Education Access & Quality:** Lower education linked to poorer health outcomes.

- **Healthcare Access & Quality:** Lack of insurance, provider shortages, culturally incompetent care.

- **Neighborhood & Built Environment:** Unsafe neighborhoods, lack of green space, poor housing conditions, lack of transportation.

- **Social & Community Context:** Social isolation, discrimination, lack of social support, civic participation.

- **Nurse's Role:**

  - **Screen & Assess:** Ask patients about potential SDOH needs (e.g., "Do you have stable housing?" "Do you worry about having enough food?" "Do you have reliable transportation to appointments?").

  - **Acknowledge Impact:** Recognize how these factors contribute to stress and mental health challenges.

  - **Refer & Collaborate:** Connect patients with community resources (food banks, housing assistance, job training, transportation services). Work closely with social workers.

  - **Advocate:** Advocate for individual patient needs and potentially for broader policy changes addressing SDOH inequities.

Case Snippet: SDOH Impact

- *Scenario:* A patient repeatedly misses therapy appointments. When the nurse explores this, the patient reveals they lack reliable transportation and sometimes have to choose between paying for the bus fare or buying food.

- *Nursing Considerations:* Recognizing transportation and food insecurity as SDOH barriers is key. The nurse collaborates with social work to explore transportation assistance programs and connect the patient with local food resources. Addressing these basic needs is essential for the patient to engage effectively in mental health treatment.

Embracing Richness and Complexity

People are not diagnoses. They are individuals shaped by their unique developmental stage, life experiences, cultural background, identity, and social circumstances. Providing truly effective mental health care requires us to look beyond the immediate symptoms and consider the whole person within their unique context. This means adapting our approach— whether communicating with a child, assessing an older adult, practicing cultural humility, providing affirming care to an LGBTQ+ individual, or addressing social barriers. It adds layers of complexity, yes, but embracing this diversity is fundamental to providing equitable, respectful, and genuinely person-centered nursing care. Finally, let us turn inward and consider how we sustain ourselves in this demanding work.

Core Learnings from This Section

- Care must be adapted across the **lifespan**. Consider developmental stage for **children/adolescents** (use play, involve family). For **older adults**, differentiate from normal aging, address polypharmacy/comorbidities, assess for depression/NCDs/suicide risk ("start low, go slow" with meds).

- Practice **Cultural Humility:** Lifelong learning, self-reflection, asking about patient beliefs/preferences, using interpreters. Avoid stereotypes.

- Provide **LGBTQ+-Affirming Care:** Use correct names/pronouns, create safe environment, understand minority stress, connect with resources.

- Address **Social Determinants of Health (SDOH):** Screen for needs (housing, food, transport), recognize impact on mental health, refer to resources, advocate.

- Person-centered care requires acknowledging and adapting to individual developmental, cultural, and social contexts.

Chapter 20 Self Care and Resilience for the Nurse

Mental health nursing offers profound rewards—witnessing recovery, building deep connections, making a tangible difference in lives marked by suffering. Yet, this work inherently exposes us to intense emotions, trauma stories, challenging behaviors, and systemic frustrations. Without conscious attention to our own well-being, the demands can lead to exhaustion, cynicism, and compromised care. Prioritizing **self-care** and cultivating **resilience** aren't luxuries in this field; they are professional necessities for sustained effectiveness, ethical practice, and personal health.

Recognizing Compassion Fatigue and Burnout

Being constantly exposed to suffering while needing to remain empathetic can take a toll. It's essential to recognize the warning signs of two related but distinct phenomena:

- **Compassion Fatigue:** Often described as "secondary traumatic stress," this results from absorbing the trauma and pain of others. It's the emotional residue of bearing witness to suffering.

  - **Symptoms:** Emotional exhaustion, reduced empathy or feeling numb, increased cynicism or irritability, difficulty separating work/personal life, intrusive thoughts/images related to patients' trauma, heightened anxiety or hypervigilance, physical symptoms (headaches, fatigue, sleep disturbance). It can feel like you've "absorbed" too much pain.

- **Burnout:** A broader state of emotional, physical, and mental exhaustion caused by prolonged exposure to workplace stressors (not just trauma exposure, but workload, lack of control, poor support, value conflicts).

- **Three Core Components:**
    1. **Emotional Exhaustion:** Feeling drained, depleted, unable to give more.
    2. **Depersonalization/Cynicism:** Developing a detached, callous, or cynical attitude towards patients, colleagues, or the job itself. Loss of idealism.
    3. **Reduced Personal Accomplishment:** Feeling ineffective, lacking achievement, doubting one's competence or the significance of one's work.

Both compassion fatigue and burnout develop over time and exist on a continuum. Early recognition allows for intervention before they become deeply entrenched. Pay attention to changes in your mood, energy levels, attitude toward work, relationships, and physical health. Be aware of these signs not just in yourself, but in your colleagues too.

Self-Assessment Checklist (Consider if these are present frequently/persistently):

- Feeling emotionally drained or exhausted after work?
- Feeling more cynical or detached from patients/work lately?
- Feeling less effective or like your work doesn't make a difference?
- Having trouble sleeping or experiencing unusual fatigue?
- Experiencing increased irritability or anger?
- Feeling numb or having difficulty feeling empathy?
- Having intrusive thoughts or images related to patient experiences?

- Dreading going to work?

- Withdrawing from social activities or relationships?

- Experiencing more frequent physical complaints (headaches, stomach issues)?

(Answering yes to several may indicate a need to prioritize self-care and seek support)

Strategies for Stress Management and Self Care

Self-care isn't just about bubble baths and vacations (though those can help!). It's about intentionally building practices into your life—both at work and outside of it—that replenish your energy and protect your well-being. Resilience isn't about being untouched by stress; it's about developing the capacity to bounce back from adversity.

Workplace Strategies:

- **Set Boundaries:**

    o **Time Boundaries:** Try to leave work on time. Avoid routinely taking work home (mentally or physically). Turn off work email notifications after hours.

    o **Task Boundaries:** Learn to say "no" or negotiate when asked to take on excessive responsibilities beyond your capacity (easier said than done, but important). Delegate when appropriate.

    o **Emotional Boundaries:** Maintain professionalism. Be empathetic but avoid over-identifying or taking on patients' problems as your own. Debrief difficult situations.

- **Take Your Breaks:** Step away from the unit during meal breaks if possible. Take short micro-breaks during the shift for deep breathing or stretching.

- **Utilize Debriefing:** Participate in formal or informal debriefing sessions after critical incidents (restraints, patient death, significant trauma exposure). Processing events as a team is crucial.

- **Seek Supportive Supervision:** Use clinical supervision to discuss challenging cases and emotional reactions (more on this below).

- **Advocate for Healthy Workplace:** Promote positive work environments, adequate staffing, manageable workloads, and access to support resources.

Personal Strategies (The SELF mnemonic can be helpful - Sleep, Exercise, Laughter/Leisure, Food):

- **Prioritize Sleep:** Aim for consistent, adequate sleep (usually 7-9 hours). Practice good sleep hygiene (dark room, cool temperature, avoid screens before bed, consistent schedule).

- **Engage in Regular Exercise:** Physical activity is a powerful stress reliever and mood booster. Find activities you enjoy (walking, running, swimming, dancing, team sports). Aim for consistency.

- **Nourish Your Body:** Eat regular, balanced meals. Stay hydrated. Limit excessive caffeine, sugar, and processed foods, which can exacerbate stress responses.

- **Practice Relaxation/Mindfulness:** Incorporate techniques like deep breathing exercises, progressive muscle relaxation, meditation, mindfulness apps, or yoga. Even 5-10 minutes daily can make a difference.

- **Cultivate Hobbies & Interests:** Engage in activities outside of nursing that bring you joy, creativity, or relaxation. Make time for things unrelated to work.

- **Maintain Social Connections:** Spend quality time with supportive friends, family, partners. Nurture relationships that replenish you. Avoid isolating yourself.

- **Set Aside "Me Time":** Schedule regular time purely for yourself, even if brief, to do something you enjoy or simply rest without obligations.

- **Practice Gratitude:** Intentionally focusing on positive aspects of life can shift perspective and build resilience. Consider keeping a gratitude journal.

- **Limit Exposure to Negativity:** Be mindful of news consumption or excessive time spent on social media if it increases stress or negativity.

- **Seek Personal Therapy:** Therapy isn't just for patients. Many nurses find it helpful for managing work stress, processing difficult experiences, and maintaining emotional health.

Key is finding what works *for you* and making it a regular, non-negotiable part of your routine.

Importance of Peer Support and Supervision

You cannot—and should not—navigate the challenges of mental health nursing alone. Connection with colleagues and guidance from experienced mentors are vital support systems.

- **Peer Support:**
  - **Shared Understanding:** Colleagues uniquely understand the day-to-day realities, frustrations, and rewards of the job.

- o Validation: Sharing experiences with peers normalizes reactions and reduces feelings of isolation ("You feel that way too? I thought it was just me!").

- o Practical Advice: Peers can offer tips, strategies, and different perspectives on managing difficult situations.

- o Emotional Release: Provides a safe space to vent frustrations or share successes with people who "get it."

- o Forms: Can be informal chats with trusted colleagues, regular team huddles/check-ins, or more structured peer support groups. *Crucial Caveat:* Ensure peer support remains professional, respects patient confidentiality, and doesn't devolve into unproductive complaining or gossip.

- **Clinical Supervision:**

  - o **What it is:** A formal, regular meeting with a designated, experienced supervisor or mentor (often an advanced practice nurse, psychologist, or seasoned RN) specifically focused on clinical practice and professional development. It's *not* the same as administrative line management.

  - o **Purpose:**

    - Discuss challenging patient cases and develop effective interventions.

    - Explore ethical dilemmas and navigate complex decisions.

- Process emotional reactions to patients and clinical situations (**countertransference**). This is a key function – understanding *why* a particular patient gets under your skin or why you feel overly protective.

- Receive feedback on clinical skills and identify learning needs.

- Develop self-awareness and professional identity.

- Prevent burnout by providing a dedicated space to process work stress.

○ **Importance:** Supervision is essential for maintaining objectivity, developing clinical judgment, managing emotional responses healthily, ensuring ethical practice, and fostering professional growth. Seek it out proactively, especially early in your career or when working in high-stress areas.

Maintaining Professional Boundaries for Personal Well being

We've discussed boundaries primarily from the perspective of patient safety and therapeutic effectiveness. But they are equally important for protecting *your own* emotional energy and preventing burnout.

- **Avoiding Over-Involvement:** Empathy is essential, but merging emotionally with patients or feeling responsible for "rescuing" them leads to exhaustion. Healthy boundaries allow you to care *for* patients without carrying their burdens *as* your own.

- **Defining Your Role:** Clearly understanding your professional role helps prevent extending yourself beyond what's appropriate or sustainable (e.g., giving out personal contact information, doing excessive favors).

- **Protecting Personal Time:** Boundaries around work hours and not bringing work stress home allow you to recharge in your personal life.

- **Preventing Manipulation:** Clear boundaries protect you from being drawn into manipulative dynamics or splitting, which are emotionally draining.

- **Self-Respect:** Maintaining professional boundaries is also an act of self-respect, valuing your own well-being alongside the patient's.

Case Snippet: Nurse Burnout & Self-Care

- *Scenario:* David, an experienced psych nurse, finds himself increasingly irritable at work, dreading his shifts, feeling like he's just going through the motions, and snapping at colleagues. He has trouble sleeping and feels constantly tired. He realizes he's been skipping lunch breaks, stopped going to the gym, and spends his evenings thinking about difficult patient cases. He recognizes signs of burnout.

- *Nursing Action (Self-Care):* David decides to take action. He commits to taking his full lunch break away from the unit daily. He restarts his gym routine 3 times a week. He makes a conscious effort to leave work thoughts at work by engaging in a hobby (listening to music) on his commute home. He talks with a trusted colleague about feeling overwhelmed. Most importantly, he schedules a meeting with his clinical supervisor to discuss his feelings of burnout and specific challenging cases that are weighing on him.

- *Outcome:* Through consistent self-care practices and utilizing supervision to process work stress, David gradually begins to feel more energetic, less irritable, and more engaged at work. He learns strategies in supervision for managing countertransference with difficult patients. He recognizes self-care and supervision aren't optional, but necessary for sustainable practice.

Sustaining the Capacity to Care

Mental health nursing is a marathon, not a sprint. The emotional labor involved requires intentional strategies to protect our own well-being. Recognizing the signs of compassion fatigue and burnout, actively engaging in diverse self-care practices, seeking support from peers, utilizing clinical supervision, and maintaining firm professional boundaries are not signs of weakness—they are hallmarks of a resilient, self-aware, and sustainable nursing professional. By caring for ourselves, we preserve our ability to provide the best possible care for those who depend on us. And with that, let's bring our journey through these essentials to a close.

Core Learnings from This Section

- Mental health nursing is rewarding but carries risks of **Compassion Fatigue** (secondary trauma) and **Burnout** (exhaustion, cynicism, ineffectiveness). Recognize the signs.

- **Proactive Self-Care is essential:** Utilize workplace strategies (breaks, boundaries, debriefing) and personal strategies (sleep, exercise, nutrition, relaxation, hobbies, social support).

- **Peer Support** provides validation and practical advice from colleagues who understand

- **Clinical Supervision** is vital for processing difficult cases, managing emotional reactions (countertransference), ethical guidance, and professional growth.

- Maintaining **Professional Boundaries** protects both the patient and the nurse's well-being, preventing over-involvement and burnout.

- Self-care and resilience are necessary professional practices for sustained effectiveness and health.

Conclusion

We have traveled together through the essential landscape of mental health nursing, from foundational concepts and communication skills to understanding specific conditions, treatments, legal/ethical frameworks, and the necessity of self-care. This guide aimed to provide a clear, simplified path—a companion to your formal education and clinical experiences, designed to build confidence and competence in this specialized field.

We explored why mental health matters, the nature of the therapeutic relationship, and the power of skilled communication. We delved into the complexities of anxiety, depression, bipolar disorder, psychosis, personality disorders, substance use, trauma, and cognitive challenges, focusing always on the key nursing priorities associated with each. We examined the tools of our trade—psychopharmacology, therapeutic modalities, the nursing process itself, and crisis management techniques. We considered the legal and ethical responsibilities that shape our practice, the importance of adapting care across the lifespan and diverse populations, and critically, the need to nurture our own resilience.

This guide, however, is just that—a guide, a starting point. The true learning in mental health nursing happens through experience, reflection, mentorship, and a commitment to lifelong professional development. Each patient encounter offers an opportunity to deepen your understanding, refine your skills, and grow both professionally and personally. Seek out experienced mentors, engage actively in clinical supervision, stay curious, and never stop learning.

The impact you can make as a mental health nurse is immense. You have the privilege of accompanying individuals during their most vulnerable moments, offering not just clinical skill, but also compassion, hope, and respect. You challenge stigma, advocate for rights, foster resilience, and facilitate recovery. It is demanding work, requiring intelligence, empathy, patience, and courage. But it is also work of profound significance, contributing immeasurably to the well-being of individuals, families, and communities.

A Final Thought

In the end, beyond the theories, the diagnoses, and the interventions, mental health nursing is fundamentally about human connection. It's about seeing the person behind the illness, hearing their unique story, and offering a steady presence in the midst of turmoil. It's about recognizing the shared humanity that links us all, understanding that mental suffering is part of the human condition, and believing in the capacity for healing and growth. Carry that understanding, that respect, and that hope into your practice, and you will truly embody the art and science of mental health nursing. Your journey is just beginning.

References

1. Agency for Healthcare Research and Quality (AHRQ), 2019. *Nonpharmacologic Versus Pharmacologic Treatment for Adult Patients With Major Depressive Disorder*. Comparative Effectiveness Review No. 218. Rockville (MD): Agency for Healthcare Research and Quality (US).

2. American Psychiatric Association, 2022. *Practice Guideline for the Treatment of Patients With Schizophrenia*. 3rd ed. Washington, DC: American Psychiatric Association Publishing.

3. Barker, P., 2001. The Tidal Model: developing an empowering, person-centred approach to recovery within psychiatric and mental health nursing. *Journal of Psychiatric and Mental Health Nursing*, 8(3), pp.233-240.

4. Beck, A.T., 2005. The current state of cognitive therapy: A 40-year retrospective. *Archives of General Psychiatry*, 62(9), pp.953-959.

5. Boyd, M.A. ed., 2020. *Psychiatric nursing: Contemporary practice*. 7th ed. Philadelphia: Wolters Kluwer. *(Note: While a book, core nursing texts are often referenced in this context)*.

6. Bradford, A., Rickwood, D., 2014. Nurses' experience of clinical supervision: a qualitative study. *Journal of Psychiatric and Mental Health Nursing*, 21(1), pp.25-33.

7. Chan, Z.C.Y., Fung, Y.L. & Chien, W.T., 2013. Bracketing in phenomenology: Only undertaken in the data collection and analysis process? *The Qualitative Report*, 18(30),

pp.1-9. *(Relevant for understanding patient experience)*.

8. Cleary, M., Deacon, M. & Jackson, D., 2011. Understanding the therapeutic relationship in mental health nursing. *Journal of Psychiatric and Mental Health Nursing*, 18(5), pp.435-440.

9. Cutcliffe, J.R. & Barker, P., 2002. Considering the care of the suicidal client and the case for 'engagement and inspiring hope' or 'observations'. *Journal of Psychiatric and Mental Health Nursing*, 9(5), pp.611-621.

10. Delgado, A., 2020. Living with bipolar disorder: strategies for managing symptoms. *Issues in Mental Health Nursing*, 41(10), pp.936-942.

11. Dziopa, F. & Ahern, K., 2011. What makes a quality therapeutic relationship in psychiatric/mental health nursing: A systematic literature review. *International Journal of Mental Health Nursing*, 20(4), pp.275-286.

12. Edward, K.L., Welch, A., 2011. The extension of the therapeutic relationship: A neglected aspect of nursing practice? *Journal of Psychiatric and Mental Health Nursing*, 18(4), pp.358-364.

13. Foster, K., Usher, K. & Drieberg, M., 2018. The role of the mental health nurse in emergency departments. *International Journal of Mental Health Nursing*, 27(1), pp.87-96.

14. Fowler, J.C., Madan, A. & Allen, J.G., 2013. Approaches to managing countertransference in the treatment of borderline personality disorder. *Psychiatric Clinics of North America*, 36(2), pp.209-224.

15. Halter, M.J., 2022. *Varcarolis' Foundations of Psychiatric-Mental Health Nursing: A Clinical Approach*. 9th ed. St.

Louis, MO: Elsevier. *(Note: Another foundational nursing text)*.

16. Happell, B., Gaskin, C.J. & Byrne, L., 2015. Clinical supervision in mental health nursing: is it maintaining quality, safety and clinical effectiveness? *Issues in Mental Health Nursing*, 36(1), pp.20-27.

17. Keltner, N.L. & Steele, D., 2019. *Psychiatric Nursing*. 8th ed. St. Louis, MO: Elsevier. *(Note: Foundational nursing text)*.

18. Linehan, M.M., 1993. *Cognitive-behavioral treatment of borderline personality disorder*. New York: Guilford Press. *(Seminal work on DBT)*.

19. Looi, J.C.L. & Sachdev, P.S., 2009. The role of the mental status examination in the era of correlation neuroimaging. *Australian & New Zealand Journal of Psychiatry*, 43(5), pp.397-406.

20. McKenna, B., O'Reilly, C. & Puri, N., 2016. Trauma informed care in inpatient mental health settings: A review of the literature. *International Journal of Mental Health Nursing*, 25(3), pp.214-226.

21. Mohr, W.K., 2010. Spiritual issues in psychiatric care. *Perspectives in Psychiatric Care*, 46(3), pp.174-183.

22. National Institute for Health and Care Excellence (NICE), 2011 (updated 2021). *Common mental health problems: identification and pathways to care*. Clinical Guideline [CG123]. London: NICE.

23. Peplau, H.E., 1952. *Interpersonal relations in nursing: A conceptual frame of reference for psychodynamic nursing*. New York: G.P. Putnam's Sons. *(Classic foundational work)*.

24. Pichot, T. & Midgley, N., 2018. The therapeutic relationship in psychodynamic psychotherapy with adolescents showing symptoms of depression: A systematic review. *Frontiers in Psychology*, 9, p.2598.

25. Richmond, M.J., Pampel, F.C., Wood, R.C., & Nunes, E.V., 2017. The impact of methamphetamine use on cognitive functioning in adolescents and young adults. *Drug and Alcohol Dependence*, 170, pp.45-54.

26. Substance Abuse and Mental Health Services Administration (SAMHSA), 2014. *SAMHSA's Concept of Trauma and Guidance for a Trauma-Informed Approach*. HHS Publication No. (SMA) 14-4884. Rockville, MD: SAMHSA.

27. Stahl, S.M., 2021. *Stahl's Essential Psychopharmacology: Neuroscientific Basis and Practical Applications*. 5th ed. Cambridge: Cambridge University Press. *(Key psychopharmacology text)*.

28. Stuart, G.W., 2021. *Principles and Practice of Psychiatric Nursing*. 12th ed. St. Louis, MO: Elsevier. *(Note: Foundational nursing text)*.

29. Tarasoff v. Regents of University of California, 17 Cal.3d 425, 551 P.2d 334, 131 Cal. Rptr. 14 (Cal. 1976). *(Landmark legal case)*.

30. Townsend, M.C., 2020. *Psychiatric Mental Health Nursing: Concepts of Care in Evidence-Based Practice*. 10th ed. Philadelphia: F.A. Davis Company. *(Note: Foundational nursing text)*.

31. World Health Organization (WHO), 2013. *Mental Health Action Plan 2013-2020*. Geneva: WHO.